THE LIVER

MONKEY PRESS

Monkey Press is named after the Monkey King in The Journey to the West, the 16th century novel by Wu Chengen. Monkey blends skill, initiative and wisdom with the spirit of freedom, irreverence and a touch of mischief.

CHINESE MEDICINE FROM THE CLASSICS

THE LIVER

Claude Larre and Elisabeth Rochat de la Vallée

transcribed and edited by Caroline Root

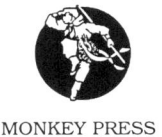

MONKEY PRESS

AcuMedic CENTRE
101-105 CAMDEN HIGH STREET
LONDON NW1 7JN
Tel: 020 7388-6704/5783
info@acumedic.com www.acumedic.com

Published by

MONKEY PRESS

www.monkeypress.com

monkey.press@virgin.net

CHINESE MEDICINE FROM THE CLASSICS: THE LIVER

Claude Larre and Elisabeth Rochat de la Vallée

© Monkey Press 1999 First edition 1994

ISBN 1 872468 07 1

Transcribed from a seminar organised by Peter Firebrace

Text Editor: Caroline Root

Production and Design: Sandra Hill

Calligraphy: Qu Lei Lei

Printed on recycled paper by RapSpiderweb

CONTENTS

FOREWORD

In many colleges of traditional Chinese medicine, both in China itself and increasingly abroad, Neijing studies are an accepted and expected part of the curriculum, since they provide the essential foundation that has been built on right up to the present day. In the Chinese Medicine from the Classics series with Claude Larre and Elisabeth Rochat de la Vallée we continue this tradition, which we hope will contribute to the growth and development of Chinese medicine in the West.

By returning to the original texts, we have the chance to study sequence and order in action, to see *how* things are presented as much as *what,* to see the context of the material as much as the material itself. So much of Chinese medicine is based on an unfolding sequence, on the flow of natural phenomena, from heaven to earth, out of winter into spring, extending into summer and retracting into autumn, to close and recharge again in winter. With the resonances of the five elements often presented now in a table form in textbooks, the interconnections can easily be lost and the internal logic broken. With the wealth of their broad knowledge of Chinese philosophy, Claude Larre and Elisabeth Rochat can restore those links, both through their patient textual analysis and through pointing out the rich cultural associations of the time. Thus medicine is no longer separated from the philosophical framework that produced it.

The liver is a powerful and dynamic organ, wide-ranging in its effects on both the free flow of *qi* and the storing and releasing of blood, connected with both motion and emotion, and the outward expression of our innate potential. The transition from the normal functioning of the liver to its pathology is graphic: obstruction, blockage, fire and wind replace the smooth harmony of budding growth. We hope that this book will go some way to bridging the gap that is sometimes apparent between the theoretical aspects of philosophy and the practical work of clinical pathology.

Peter Firebrace, London 1994

FOREWORD TO THE SECOND EDITION

This new edition of The Liver has been re-edited and formatted with the Chinese characters inserted in the text. The value of the teachings has not diminished with time. The insights and understandings presented by the authors continue to illuminate the theory and practise of Chinese medicine in the West. Indeed as Father Larre's advancing age has prevented him from travelling, this series of seminars, published as Chinese Medicine from the Classics, is a testament to the authentic and eloquent voice of one of the most significant teachers of Chinese philosophy in recent decades.

Caroline Root and Sandra Hill, Rhodes 1999

THE LIVER

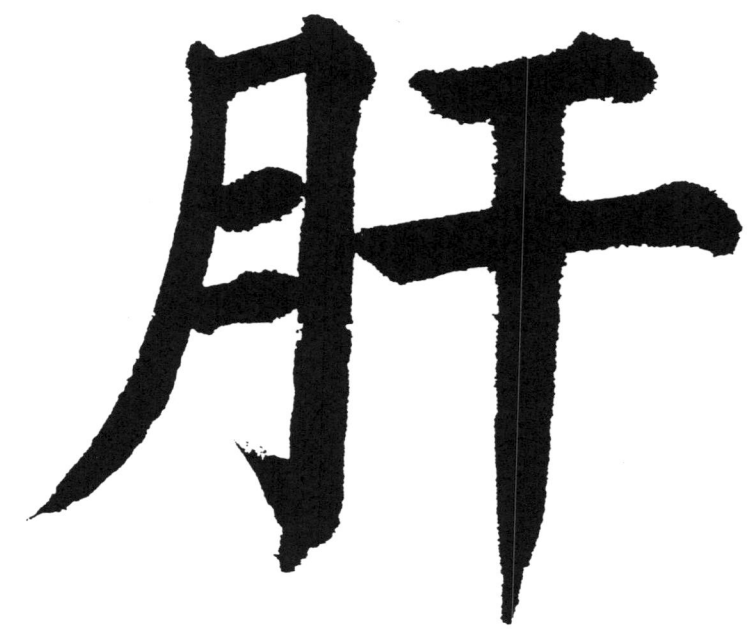

The Liver, *gan*

INTRODUCTION

Peter Firebrace: I would like to welcome Father Larre and Elisabeth Rochat de la Vallée from the European School of Acupuncture. After our last seminar covering in broad outline the twelve internal organs, we are now going to go into detail on the liver and gallbladder. If you go back directly to the Chinese texts, the strokes which make up a character seem to give a direct insight into the energetic impulses behind the fundamental concepts of Chinese medicine. By working through the Nei jing, especially the early chapters where these characters are put in a certain sequence to show the kind of movements that represent life and what happens when that is disturbed, you have a very clear perception and expression of things which is useful to us as acupuncturists. We are fortunate to have Father Larre and Elisabeth not only as translators but also as commentators. A translation is too short, it needs expanding in a commentary.

Claude Larre: I have no need to say how pleased we are to come back to London for a continuation of the work we have been doing in Oxford for the past four years. The trouble with us being French is that we do not speak enough English. But in a way that may be an advantage since it means you are obliged to pay more attention to what is said. You have to make your own translation, not from the Chinese but from that sort of half English to pure English. We ourselves have to make a more complicated journey from the Chinese text, which is not only Chinese but classical Chinese, and not only classical Chinese but classical Chinese intended to convey a lot of information on life and on normal and pathological ways of life. From that we come not to a translation but to some sort of intuition or comprehension of what the text means or wants to convey, all the time being very much aware that there is not just one way of apprehending life.

I feel that these seminars will be very helpful, not only for a theoretical basis but also for practice. Elisabeth has a very broad understanding of the Chinese classics, she knows when things are and she even knows when things are not. I personally do not know very much about acupuncture theory, but I know more about the larger setting of the so-called Chinese medical books within the broader framework of classical thought and specifically the Zhuang zi, the Lao zi, the Huainan zi and the other books which are usually the ultimate references for any Chinese medical text. The differences are not those between schools of thought, but rather what is appropriate for a specific medical case where the needle is called for, not a brush or a government. There is no difference in the way the universe is ruled and how my own individual body, mind and spirit might be.

The programme today is on the liver and gallbladder. As everybody knows there must always be a teaching on a pair of so-called meridians since one is the leading factor and the other is on another level helping the first. There is some sort of subordination and co-operation, one is principally in charge, but is unable to make the function work properly without the other. This is seen everywhere, but specifically in Zhuang zi chapter 2 where something is said of the way the universe moves inside and outside of oneself. Looking from that point of view we are able to see that there is no pronouncement on human life which is not at the same time a pronouncement of the universal way, what we call *dao* (道), as in the Dao de jing, or what we call virtue, *de* (德) which is very close to the *dao*.

Because an individual is a person who is made and sustained and destroyed by the universe itself, we feel that it is impossible to make a presentation of just the liver or the gallbladder, even in the Chinese way; we really have to take a view of all life, and we know that there are at least five aspects through which life is seen, as is distinctly stated in Su wen chapter 5. If I feel that the heart is the supreme governor I am fearful that the beating of my heart may stop and that the sovereign will then be without either kingdom or power. So usually I feel that as long as my heart is beating correctly and strongly enough I am in good health. But at the same time if I am a woman of about 49 or a man of about 64, I feel the lack of some sort of kidney energy, and I am no longer in a position, broadly speaking, to give the surplus of my life outside myself and create another life. So turning from the role of heart to the role of kidneys I hesitate and say maybe it is not the heart which is so important? The heart is the sovereign but the true power ascends in myself and is ready to expand outwards, so that is the power of the kidneys. But sitting beside the bed of a dying person I see that if the breath stops then life will stop, so I may have the feeling that life is not so much a question of the kidneys or the heart but of breathing and the lungs.

Looking at a plant I see that the first foliage is a very small green blade coming forth from the ground, giving the impression of life. Dropping the more complicated expressions of life, animal, vegetable or human, and just concentrating on the impulse of life which is seen through the expansion from green blade to plant to tree, with many branches and much foliage, then maybe all life is just constructed on this same principle. The final expression of life is just the combination of the more essential functions related to the less noble functions, all working together to bring forth and sustain life, and make it radiate. That is a concept of life. So we are not dismissing the lung or the heart or the kidneys, but today we will just take the aspect of life which is represented as wood within the five elements, the muscular forces (*jin* 筋) within the body actions, and the liver within the organs. We are able to see this fibre which makes the wood able to expand and extend, working in the universe through the colour green and through all the muscular forces.

First, to give a broad presentation we will make reference to the classical texts. This is not a luxury or something just for the specialist. It is something for everybody. From the theoretical side it is impossible to fully understand anything systematically if you do not refer to the texts. If you do not know Chinese, you cannot understand everything from just reading a translation. Our discussion and presentation are an effort to give you access to the Chinese texts, because we take for granted that you do not know and do not want to learn Chinese! We have been studying these texts for years, and our position is that it is not only possible but necessary to convey the spirit and the organizational structure of the text. So this is a sort of general plea, not for your attention, but for your willingness to perceive what stands behind what is said. We do not summarize or make a résumé of anything in order to replace what is said by the Chinese by what we feel should be said. Many conflicts between different schools arise just because they lack the ability or even the desire to go to where the tradition has lain for centuries and centuries. There is no need to say that one text from the Ming Dynasty contradicts another from the Song Dynasty, or that the Song Dynasty so greatly changed the outlook of the Chinese that it is no longer the same thing as was commented upon during the Tang Dynasty. Not to mention the more original texts of the Han Dynasty or to take into account that what is written has been spoken not for centuries but for millennia.

NEI JING TEXTS

SU WEN CHAPTER 8

Claude Larre: Let us turn to the presentation in Su wen chapter 8 where the charges (*guan* 官) are described and named, and then go through the first chapters of the Nei jing and see how the liver is presented. The name of chapter 8 is 'The Secret Treatise of the Spiritual Orchid'. It starts with a question from Huang di, and he asks to be instructed on the relative charges and ranks of the 12 *zang* (臟). The celestial master, Qi Bo, replies 'What a vast question! If you will allow me, let us go through it all.' The specific charges of the liver and gallbladder are as follows:

> *The liver holds the office of general of the armed forces.*
> *Assessment of circumstances and conception of plans*
> *stem from it.*

*The gallbladder is responsible for what is just and exact.
Determination and decision stem from it.*

This Treatise is secret and is kept in a special place in the
Imperial palace library called the Spiritual Orchid, *ling lan*
(靈 蘭). We understand from this name that the essence of
life is preserved through the various charges of the *zang fu*
(臟 府). If the Treatise is secret it is just because it can be
dangerous to let everyone know secrets if they are not able
to act in accordance with the knowledge. In a way this is
right, because it is never good to throw pearls to swine. But
you may ask 'Who are swine and who are not?' That is
something we do not know, and the feeling of a democracy
is that we have to give the best to the worst, and that it is
right to disseminate knowledge. But if you print what is
secret for public use then it is necessarily different, and
what is printed is never what was sought after. Behind
every thought is observation and the reflection of mind and
spirit on what has been observed. So a good way to teach
pathology is to give all the information through observations
of the way the liver and gallbladder function as they should,
and it is only when something goes astray or when something
is wrong that we see clearly what should be. When everything
goes as it should it is so silent, so invisible and so secret
that it is nearly impossible to understand what it is about.
So it is through pathology that we have clues to normality.

In the first 12 chapters of the Su wen and the Ling shu

where the general functions and outlook on life are given, normality and pathology are presented at the same time. It usually starts with normality and then alludes to the pathology. But the more you proceed through the 81 chapters of the Nei jing, the Ling shu or the Nan jing, the more it is the pathology which is described since these books were intended to help people cure diseases. There may sometimes seem a slight contradiction at points between the emphasis on the expansion of life, with the green and the wood and the foliage, and the defence of life aspect found in Su wen chapter 8 which talks of the general commanding the armed forces with the gallbladder assisting in decision making. This is an open question.

SU WEN CHAPTER 2

The three months of spring
are called spring forth and display.
Heaven and earth together produce life,
and the 10,000 beings are invigorated.

At night one goes to bed, at dawn one gets up.
One paces in the courtyard with great strides,
hair loose, body relaxed, exerting the will for life,
to give life and not to kill, to give and not to take,
to reward and not to punish.

This is the way that is proper to the qi of spring,
which thus corresponds
to the maintaining of the production of life.

To go against this current would injure the liver,
causing illnesses in the summer due to cold,
through an insufficient contribution to growth.

SU WEN CHAPTER 2

Claude Larre: Su wen chapter 2 might be titled 'A Distribution of Life through the Four Seasons'. It is all about the process of explosion, expansion, exhaustion and contraction, as seen throughout the year. Spring is like a spring, it makes a movement, while summer conserves the same movement and gives it stability. You take your vacation in summer not because you are tired but because it is time to let the *qi* go freely outside. Then at a certain moment when the general condition of the universe is no longer in the ascent, when the *yang* (陽) has given most of its expansion, the other side of life, the *yin* (陰), has to take its turn being dominant and you have autumn. Autumn is somewhat strange in that sometimes it is closer to summer and sometimes closer to winter, but usually autumn is the time when we amass, harvest and hoard things awaiting winter. Then we have to close the doors, take care of our condition, draw from the reserves we have collected during the autumn and quietly wait for the renewal of life in ourselves and in nature at large. This cycle is so important that there is no way we can treat people ignoring the season in which the treatment is given.

So what about the liver in relation to this question of the four seasons? The text says:

The three months of spring
are called spring forth and display

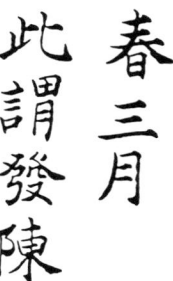

The Chinese will often use an expression made of two characters in order to clearly indicate the beginning of the process, and also to demonstrate the tendency of the process. So spring is a time when life is sprouting. The character *fa* (發), to spring forth, is very expressive. The upper part is more or less the crust of the earth, or some sense of opposition. Below is a bow and arrow and an archer. This is the way in which Chinese characters represent the condition of the universe when life is ready to come forth, to spring up and to sprout. There is a tension in that movement as in a drawn bow. The initiative for life is seen to be related to the power of heaven, but the actual manifestation of life is seen on the earth. There is an earthly effect that is springing everywhere, so it expands as much as it springs, and this is taken as being related to earth. Since every one of the 10,000 beings is ruled by the combination of heavenly and earthly energy, it is normal that I should feel heaven in myself and that I should want to accompany the movement with some sort of horizontal extension. I get up and I expand,

and that is spring. This is the production of life. Heaven and earth together produce life, and life having been produced the movement goes on to maintain and sustain it. So the text says:

> *Heaven and earth together produce life and the 10,000 beings are invigorated.*

The text continues:

> *At night one goes to bed, at dawn one gets up. One paces about in the courtyard with great strides, hair loose, body relaxed, exerting the will for life; to give life and not to kill, to give and not to take, to reward and not to punish. This is the way that is proper to the qi of spring which thus corresponds to the maintaining of the production of life.*

> *To go against this current would injure the liver, causing illnesses in the summer due to cold through an insufficient contribution to growth.*

At this point the liver is mentioned for the first time in the text. So an insufficient contribution to growth has something to do with the state of the liver, and an excessive contribution to growth is also a state which has to be dispersed in order that the harmony of the other functions is kept well. For example, if you give too much to someone in a family, perhaps the others will start to press their demands; it is never good to give too much without taking care of the effect on the general balance and harmony. If you feel very excited in spring you may tolerate it because it is in the nature of the *qi* (氣) at that time, but if you feel very excited in other seasons then you endanger other functions. A little excitement is normal because nothing can be so regulated that it stands still, and it depends on what sort of person and age you are, and also what sort of acupuncturist you meet with!

Elisabeth Rochat: In Su wen chapter 2 we can find all the great principles of the physiology and pathology of the liver. The three months of spring which are described as springing up, spreading out and developing, extend all the effects connected with the function of the liver, being at the beginning of all movement. This function is described as making things flow or propagating, *shu xie* (疏 泄). In the liver it is the vital impulse which is necessary for the manifestation of life. And this aspect of being the manifestation of a source of life or a strength of life is the answer to Father Larre's question as to why the liver is both the general of the armed forces and this principle of life. The liver is a manifestation of strength and the great and visible impulse of life. In the natural world or in the universe this is the power of spring and of vegetation in the spring when flowers and plants just spread out on the earth. Within society this manifests most clearly in the armed forces.

Obviously this strength is based on the kidneys. In Su wen chapter 2 we find it said in the section describing the three months of winter that if we go against the current proper to the *qi* of winter, then we injure the kidneys causing a weakening in springtime which is exactly like an impotence, or a lack of the power of life. This is the connection between the kidneys and the liver.

The same thing has already appeared in the first chapter of the Su wen, because in that chapter very few organs appear, just the kidneys, liver and heart. The heart appears as the centre of human life and has to be peaceful and empty like a void, so that all circulation can take place. In the period of reproductive life everything is stated with reference to the kidney *qi*. Then, at the end of the time when a man has the power to produce another life with his own, the liver is mentioned. The liver *qi* declines because its basis lies in the kidneys, and as their power decreases you do not have the strength to draw back the bow and fire the arrow. This image is found in the first ideogram we mentioned when talking of the three months of spring, *fa* (發).

We can find this connection between the kidneys as the base, and the liver as a spreading out effect in many circumstances. For example in the relation between muscular forces and bones. The muscular forces make a connection between the bones and the flesh in order to allow movement. This enables us to see not the interior deep strength of the kidneys but the visible movement of the whole body. During springtime heaven and earth together produce life, and this is the same as the junction through the liver of *yin* and *yang*, blood and *qi*. We will see this later, but there are two sides of the liver: the substance which is in the blood and *yin*, and the effect produced, which is the *qi*. This is the *yang* force which is the strength of the liver to spread out and circulate. Each of the organs has this conjunction of *yin* and *yang* but in different ways.

Heaven and earth together
produce life
and the 10,000 beings
are invigorated

萬物以榮　天地俱生

In the character for invigorated (*rong* 榮) we can find the ideogram for wood (木). Above are two fires and beneath there is a roof and wood. This is very similar to the ideogram for the nutritive *qi* (*ying* 營). In *ying* the idea is to bring together all the elements which are necessary to build the body and mind and so on. There is a structure which is something like a military camp or a palace or some kind of building. *Ying* is the movement of structuration, of construction and building, while *rong* is the movement of making the sap rise to invigorate the life of plants and trees.

Rong is also the name of one of the series of five element command points. Naturally one function of the liver is to invigorate all the body through the distribution and regulation of the quantity of blood, and to invigorate the muscular forces.

At night one goes to bed
at dawn one gets up

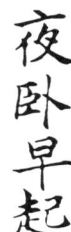

This follows the natural movement of the *qi* inside and outside, the regulation of waking and sleeping, of moving and ceasing to move.

One paces about in the courtyard
with great strides,
hair loose, body relaxed,
exerting the will for life

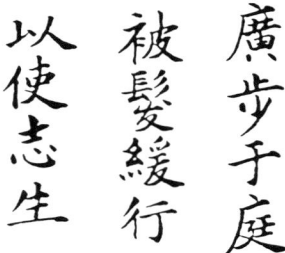

This is the beginning of motion after the hibernation of winter. The muscular forces must be unleashed again. The *qi* must circulate freely now, and go up to the top of the body which is the end of the liver meridian. You will remember that it is the only *yin* meridian which has a pathway through the head to the summit and the meeting point of all the *yang qi*.

Claude Larre: Confucius, in every description of him, is said to have had a sort of depression in the skin and bone at the top of his head in order to collect all the *yang*. It is the point of the 100 meetings, *bai hui* (百 會), or the meeting place of the 100 animating powers. Speaking of 100 always implies the full expanse or totality of something.

Elisabeth Rochat: Because Confucius was the ideal of wisdom, some special connection with the strength of the kidneys had to be manifest. This depression at the top of the head was to collect the benevolent influences coming from above in the same way that water is collected in a hollow or a pond. The great Emperor Shun had two pupils in each eye because he could see everything and show the radiance of life from his own interior light and spirit. Lao zi had big ears resting on his shoulders to collect the sounds of the world. The wisdom of Lao zi was so great that it strained the forces of the kidneys which was why the ears, the special orifices of the kidneys, were especially developed.

During spring and during this movement in the universe, which in a human being is called the liver, the muscular forces and all the body have to begin to move. But you have to take care not to go too far and not to get too tired. For this reason we find in the pathology this tiredness. The liver has responsibility for the quality and quantity of movement, for the quantity of blood, and for the mastery of the muscular forces. Also, through the spirit of the liver there is the decision and determining of where and when to stop. The hair must be loose, the body relaxed without being too tired - because above all the great function of the liver is to make the *qi* circulate well. Expressing the will for life has the same meaning as the expansion of life. This is expansion, not in the same way that the heart or spleen expands, but expansion as an impulse with an upward direction. It is an exploding impulse. It is a pushing of life, pushing up and out, like the ideogram *sheng* (生). If we go against this current we will injure the liver, and in summer we will have illnesses due to cold, and if not exactly illnesses then some kind of blockage in growing upwards. It is like a plant which has caught the frost, and then never grows properly because the *qi* can never circulate and penetrate everywhere as it should. For this reason in the pathology of the liver we find all kinds of blockages in the circulation of *qi*, and the balance between the blood that is stored and reconstituted in the liver and the *qi* of the liver which must be very well preserved all the time.

SU WEN CHAPTER 4

The natural green aspect of the eastern quarter
penetrates and spreads to the liver.
It opens its orifice at the eye,
it stores the essences in the liver.
Its disturbance is indicated by starting and trembling,
its taste is acid, its own species is grass and wood,
its domestic animal is the cock, its cereal is wheat.

Corresponding to the four seasons,
in the heights it is the planet Jupiter.
Consequently the qi of spring is in the head.
Its note is the note jue, its number is eight.
Consequently its illness is seen in the muscular forces.
Its smell is rancid.

SU WEN CHAPTER 4

Claude Larre: Let us turn to chapter 4. Chapter 2 is well known for its presentation of the four seasons, and the development of what makes spring the spring, summer the summer, autumn the autumn and winter the winter. The Chinese use analogy as a principle for understanding the deepest meaning of their ways of thinking about life. They observe life, but they do not just create an idea out of it. They use their minds in such a way that they can give different names to a particular feeling according to the different phenomena which are manifest in resonance with it. Chapter 4 starts with the east which is the spring, and with the aspect or colour, *se* (色).

The natural green aspect
of the eastern quarter
penetrates and spreads to the liver

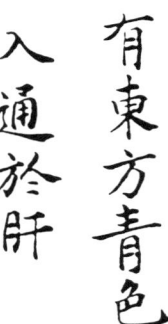

The character *se* (色) is usually translated as 'colour', but what is colour? Colour is the aspect, and the visible aspect of nature in the spring is a sort of green. Behind this impression there is the reality of the vision before the colour is declared, and that is the aspect. We make a very profound distinction between the aspect of things and the colour they have.

The chapter goes on with the division of space into four or five regions. If we are talking of four then it is east, west, north and south. If we are talking of five then it is east, west, north, south and a central region. When we have to enter into the movement of life the addition of the centre is necessary. The same is true with time. We may oppose one season with another, spring and autumn, winter and summer. Spring and autumn are transitional periods of time, and winter and summer are a confirmation of that initial transition. In this way we only need the distribution of time through four seasons. But if we want to look at the interplay of one season with another, an additional season is necessary to see how one season progresses, contradicts or glides into another, having some kind of dominance or recession.

We start with what we call a quadrant. A quadrant is a division by four, a division of space. The east is a portion of space, if it were only a direction we would call it the eastern direction.

Elisabeth Rochat: The ideograms *ru tong* (入 通) are translated 'it penetrates and spreads'. *Tong* (通) is to be in vital communication with, to receive *qi* from heaven or from something which constitutes the structure of the thing. *Tong* is vital communication which is absolutely free and without blockage. It communicates the virtue of the thing which is in relationship with something else at the very highest level. For instance, all living beings are in a relationship with the *qi* of heaven in order to be alive and remain alive. This is at the most general level, but the first particular level of the dissemination of *qi* through time and space makes the eastern quadrant and the four seasons.

Claude Larre: If it were only the impression of colour seen by your eye it could not be said to penetrate. It is a specific quality of *qi* of which the aspect is *qing* (青), the natural green, and that quality of *qi* penetrates and spreads to the liver. You see then the immense difference of approach between what you see and what is acting. Chapter 4 demonstrates what the *qi* related to this eastern quadrant is doing.

It opens its orifice at the eye

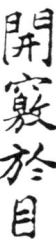

The liver itself is not visible to us deep within the body, but if something can penetrate it, it has to have an opening on the exterior part of the body. Likewise if something has to move from your own interior self outwards, then it needs some sort of orifice to get out. The eye is the orifice corresponding to the liver.

'Open' in Chinese has two important and different meanings. One is just to open, and the other is to make something move, for example like starting a car. When you say in Chinese 'I open my car' you mean I am starting the engine. Therefore, to open or to have an opening implies a function, not just a location of the orifice. The meaning of open is then the connection between the interior and the exterior, or from the exterior to the interior, all of which takes place via the eye.

Elisabeth Rochat: The first part of the text is just a penetration, a profusion of *qi*, and the certain quality of *qi* which constitutes the liver, and then finally at the end of this movement is the eye. It is the extension of this *qi* of the eastern quarter, which communicates life in the form of the liver within the human body, and which going further and further results in the eye. The eye is the highest orifice, and has a very intimate relationship with the brain. Through the eyes a human being can project far away, with a powerful look, and with radiance. The orifice is just the continuation of this movement from the liver, and through the liver out to the exterior world.

Claude Larre: I would like to clarify a point. Since we are adults we have a body and we have eyes, and we talk of bodies and eyes from our standpoint. But actually that is not the case in the text. There we find just what there is. We start from the most pure and indistinct aspect of what exists. As far as life is concerned it is to be found first in the eastern quarter or quadrant. From that you build, or you look at the self-building of different beings, and it happens that the sort of light which is emitted through the power of life coming from what we call the liver, forms and acts in a way which finally results in the physical eye which you all know. So it is not saying that the eye is made from this and that, it is the reverse. Things are, and they evolve, and they come to that point at which it is safe to call that function 'liver', whatever liver might be. And this function has a relationship to the external world and a relationship to myself which is identical to the self of the universe.

It is very important not to make the Chinese think and talk as we do. We just need to follow the movement of the text which is already there. This is the reason why we insist on knowing certain characters, and knowing the connection from one character to another. If we do not enter through that door everything will be accommodated to our way of thinking and never be like the Chinese text.

It stores the essences in the liver

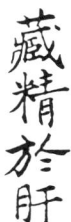

It is proper to the *zang* (臟) to store or treasure. The liver stores essences, *jing* (精), but what sort of essences? In fact all kinds of essences may go to the liver; essences will always go where they belong, and nothing is stored but the purest, since what is not pure causes problems and is rejected. If it is not rejected then the liver is endangered. The proper place, the proper time and the proper thing are necessary for the upkeep of life.

Elisabeth Rochat: The second part of the text begins 'it stores the essences in the liver'. So the liver is now able to become a centre of structuration because it fulfils its responsibility as a *zang* storing essences. When the liver forms a structure in the body, it is able to express this structure as muscular forces. Muscular forces (*jin* 筋) are similar to the liver or wood or plants because they can bend and stretch and then straighten out. This is the great characteristic of the wood element, a kind of firmness together with flexibility. Muscular forces, which are not flesh but are the link and the connection between flesh and bones, are exactly like vegetation or wood, and the ideogram *jin* (筋) is actually made with the bamboo character along with the radicals for flesh and strength. Bamboo is very firm, yet flexible and useful. *Jin* is ordinarily translated as muscular forces or muscles or tendons, and there is the expression *jing jin* (經 筋), the muscular meridians, which has the same character. There is a link between bones and flesh through the motion of muscular forces which we call movements. The wind is also characterised by this kind of beginning of movement, like the leaves of a tree in a breeze. This is a good movement for life, for the liver and for the muscular forces, because the liver gives the impulse to make the *qi* circulate well and the blood to be well nourished.

Claude Larre: With reference to the character *jin* I would remind you that each time you see a character you have to understand the meaning on two levels. There are tendons which you are able to see when you cut the body open, but it is not only that physical aspect which is being referred to, it is rather the fact that something has been able to produce this physical form which we call a tendon. The meaning is always the tangible, physical, material aspect which makes a tendon something you understand, but at the same time the living body needs inspiration so as not to be dead flesh but to be real and acting.

All this is understood as a 'fusion', as how the heavenly power meets the earthly in order to produce a tendon, a function and the thing which permits the function to exist. Whenever a part of the body is alluded to you must recall in your mind the double aspect of heaven and earth, and the crossing at which human life is possible. So the composition of a character with bamboo, flesh and strength is more than a physical description, and it is the combination of the three parts which makes this bending and stretching of life possible. If you look at that from the point of view of earth then the tendon is not the liver, if you look at it from the point of view of heaven the tendon and the liver are the same. If you look at it from the point of view of the crossing of heaven and earth then the tendon comes from the liver and the liver is for the tendon. This sort of very simple logic has to be kept in mind in order that you do not stumble on the French or English words used to convey the meaning of the Chinese text.

Its disturbance is indicated
by starting and trembling

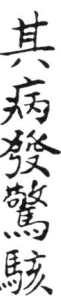

After the normal state of a healthy man is described you have the disorder. The disturbance in the liver is indicated by something visible - starting and trembling. The character for starting, *jing* (驚), is made with the ideogram for horse, *ma* (馬), underneath. Horses are very sensitive, and when you move a horse you have to speak to it and stroke its body so that it will not be surprised. Starting is the most inner feeling at the beginning of the movement of a horse. Trembling is the most external effect of this starting, just as in a car you start the engine and the engine trembles within the body of the car and there is a shaking movement. This is an exact description of what happens when the essences which are stored or hoarded in the liver with its special combination of *qi* and blood, are set in motion. The character for trembling, *hai* (駭), is also made with the horse radical. So the horse is very interesting. Whenever you see a horse walking around in a medical text you can be sure that it is something to do with fear and surprise.

Elisabeth Rochat: When the quality of movement of the liver is disturbed we have a lot of illness with trembling, and this is very important in the pathology of the liver.

Its taste is acid

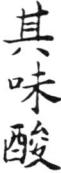

Claude Larre: As with the question of aspect and colour, there is a similar situation with taste. When you taste good wine you have the feeling on your tongue and palate, and even in your mind, that it is a really good burgundy or whatever. French wines are just a little better than others of course! What you have is the impression on your tongue. This is built from an important combination of structures which mean that the sun has been captured by the foliage of the vine, and has continued under the special conditions of the cellar to produce the taste.

But when the Chinese are talking of the five tastes they are talking primarily of what constitutes the basis for your appreciation of a taste: the colour, the notes, the perfume, the savour. All that is understood in Chinese as two different aspects. One is the thing itself, and the other is the effect of that thing on your own organs and sense organs.

Elisabeth Rochat: As Father Larre said taste is a way of testing the internal structure of something. An internal structure is like the essence, it is a very deep living component of something, which can show an aspect like natural green or a taste like acid.

Its own species is grass and wood

其
類
草
木

You can note that the Chinese text in this chapter does not just say wood but 'grass and wood', all vegetation with its fibrous aspect.

Its domestic animal is the cock

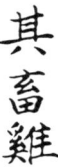

其
畜
雞

Claude Larre: The corresponding species to grass and wood in the animal kingdom is the cock. The cock is full of animation, with his red crest and his demeanour in the courtyard. All that is the external sign of the special energy which in the animal kingdom makes him the king, and related to the liver.

Elisabeth Rochat: There is also a very classical connotation because we find the cock in the Yi jing, the Book of Change. A cock is not only a proud and haughty animal but also the one which carefully chooses its food, pecking on the ground for seeds. This is the double aspect of the liver which is the general of the armed forces but which also has the function of conceiving of plans and assessing circumstances, choosing very carefully and selecting a good path to follow.

Its cereal is wheat

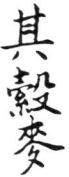

This is very difficult to understand. Some classical commentators say it is because wheat ripens early, like the spring, but really I do not know.

Corresponding to the four seasons,
in the heights it is the planet Jupiter

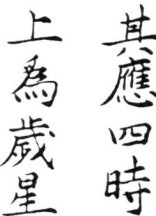

In the second part of this text we are no longer in space or in structure. We are now in the cycle of time, and in this cycle there is a model of time in the form of five planets. Above us the circulation and permutation of these planets is like the ideal pattern for all the cycles of time on earth, not only seasons but all cycles of time inside the body, throughout a lifetime.

The five *qi* in heaven form the five planets which are the model for all cycles, seen on earth as the five elements. The five planets are the visible aspect of the quality of influences coming from above. According to the configuration of the five planets in the different months and years, we may know how heaven is giving its orientation to life.

Claude Larre: The planet related to the eastern quadrant is Jupiter. The planets move in a different way from a constellation of stars. In order to be complete and to observe life we have to observe the sky, and to make a place for the five planets. The trouble is that there are more than five, but they do not care! They are only concerned with the planets which enter the classification!

Consequently
the qi of spring is in the head

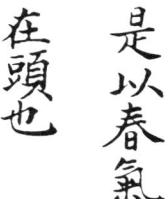

Coming to the position of the *qi* of spring, since everything is rising up, in a man we come to the head. The liver *qi* goes everywhere. There is an ascending motion for expansion and extension, and it goes to the highest place. So it is said that the *qi* of the spring is in the head, and there is a lot of pathology concerned with the head and with the connection of the head with the trunk.

Its note is the note jue

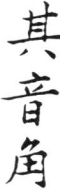

The note is not the sound, it is not what you hear, but rather the specific organization towards hearing which precedes what you hear. When I bang something you hear the sound, and the sound is under the control of a certain note. If you change the instrument you change the sound but you may play the same note. It proves that there is a difference between the note and the sound.

Elisabeth Rochat: The *qi* of this vibration is the same in quality as the note *jue* (角), and it has a corresponding echo in the quality of *qi* in the liver and in all those movements represented by the *jin* (筋). We know from the Book of Rites, Liji Yueji, what the quality of each note is:

> *There is an intimate relationship between the third note, jue, and the people. If the third note is defective, the sound is sad and the people are discontented.*

When this note is well played, at the right time and in the right place it makes people happy, full of the joy of life, and the upsurging of this life. If not the result is sadness.

Claude Larre: This needs some comment. When you are playing music it is impossible to only play that note in spring and another note in summer and so on. You have to understand that the text is not referring to music as such, but something different. It means that if you transfer that which is the liver to a sound in the order of notes, the proper note is *jue*. And if you play this note in the springtime, you will fully understand what spring is and what music is. It does not mean that you do not hear the other notes. It is just a way of singling out one note which corresponds to the state of *qi* constituting the universe and your own liver in all its functions.

Thus you can receive the true feeling of the exact connotation between the universe and sound, just as when you see the colour natural green in the spring you do not have the same feeling as when you see it in the autumn. You may have green plants in your house all year but when you see them in springtime you understand what these plants actually are.

This adjustment of notes and colours to the universe as represented both inside and outside yourself gives you the proper references for the distribution of life. Actually, in the course of time, in different spaces, all of it is mixed, and there are places where spring comes just at the time when you are expecting autumn. But that is all contingent. The important thing is to know how everything is built according to a very strict network of forces, of *qi*. We do not speak of 'energy' in the European School of Acupuncture. Energy is only the *yang* aspect of this character, and would be to misunderstand the general and very well balanced view of *dao* (道) in the universe.

Its number is eight

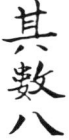

Eight may be explained in different ways. My feeling is that it is the number of the winds. There are eight winds, and there are eight winds because there are four directions which permit the subdivision of the four into eight, just to indicate some sort of movement. The eight winds are not a static division of winds. They are the representation of the movement proper to the atmosphere between heaven and earth, which is so important because it is the cause of so many diseases.

Elisabeth Rochat: In Su wen chapter 4 each organ has a special number between five and nine. Eight is three plus five. Five is the first achievement. There is a first set of numbers from one to five, and each one is attributed to an element. According to the fundamental treatise the Hong fan, one is the number of water, because water is the ancestor of all living beings, two is for fire because fire comes to mix with water and to make the kind of hot liquid which is a quality of life, three is the number of wood, four of metal and five of earth.

One and water are the same thing, like the sea and the mystery of the deep ocean. It is a reservoir of life. Through fire life can then appear, so fire is two. We also know that there are two sides of fire: ministerial fire and imperial fire. Three is the number of wood, and also the number of *qi*. Life appears between water and fire, between heaven and earth and through *qi*. Four is the number of the earth, and the earth gives all forms and shapes. Perhaps metal is the element that must be in a very strong, concentrated shape? Metal is the concentration in earth.

Claude Larre: Earth is never simply earth, it is always a mixture as there are so many things which make up humus. But gold is gold, silver is silver and lead is lead. When it is pure it is difficult to divide because it is pressed into itself. Liquid has no specific form, fire is always expanding and rising up, and wood is animated by some sort of vibration. Metal is different from these, but similar to earth. The contrast with earth is that it is pure and made only of itself. It is like one part of earth. The other aspect of earth is that being divided it is made up of everything else like some permutation of all *qi* put together.

Elisabeth Rochat: For this reason five, or earth, is the place of all exchanges. If we add this number of exchange and permutation to the other numbers we get a second series: six for water, seven for fire, eight for wood, nine for metal and ten for earth.

Question: Does the explanation for these numbers come

from the Nei jing or do you take it from the Yi jing?

Elisabeth Rochat: From the Hong fan, which is a treatise in the Shi jing, the Book of History, from the Yi jing and from the commentators who write on these books. One thing is repeated by all commentators: this first series of numbers is for giving life, in order to write the notes of different *qi* which can make life. The second series is for the work of life to achieve and to compenetrate and compose all the elements in order to perfect something which was only in its beginning in the first series.

Claude Larre: The first series is more the potential of things, and the second is more the actual being. The actual being is made from this origin when it is worked on by earth. There is nothing actual which does not come out of the earth. It is the same as the difference between the stomach and what exists before the stomach. The stomach is the place where each life may be restored through the action of the essences which enter and remain there for transformation. The stomach is not a primitive potentiality of life, it is the actual place where life is restored. So we always have to stay within the Chinese frame of life, whether it is a medical book, a painting or philosophy at large. We always have to take into account that sometimes they may be talking of things with a specificity but they are not actual things, and sometimes they are talking of an individual thing or being. You have to move from above to below. In heaven there are just the so-called images of things, while the actual things have to be drawn to earth and come forth there.

To summarize this, there are two levels of consideration. The first series of numbers is the potential of a thing, and if you want to understand things in their potential you have to go through one, two, three, four and five. That is the level of heaven. But when you come to actual beings, actual beings spring from the earth, so the second series is five plus one, two, three, four and five. Since ten and one are the same thing in the mind we sometimes just stop at nine, which is the reason why they often do not talk of ten but stop at nine.

Elisabeth Rochat: If an element has an odd number in the first series it has an even number in the second. This is transformation by the action of the permutation of *qi* through earth. Water, at the level of creation and production, was the unity, one, the first. It penetrated all things, including the depths of earth. But at the number six it is like a structuration through *yin* and through all liquids and essential body fluids. The fire, which at the level of two is like a condition of life after water, is now, in the number seven, like a spreading out of life, with communication and with tension. Wood, which was with the number of *qi*, three, is now with the number of the winds, eight, which is the occupation of space through *qi* like wind. So you can see that there is some equation in this presentation of element, number and organ.

Consequently its illness
is seen in the muscular forces

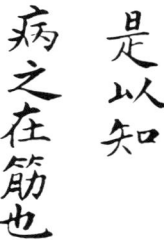

Claude Larre: As we saw earlier there is a strict connection between the constitution of the muscular forces, *jin* (筋), and wood. Looking at wood you see it as muscular forces, and looking at muscular forces you see them as made up of vibrating fibres, expanding, stretching and bending just as wood does. But since that involves blood and *qi*, if we do not have roots the variety of motion is much bigger. However, there is this similarity between mankind and plants, and human beings are just walking plants.

Its smell is rancid

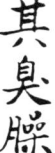

The important thing about this presentation in chapter 4 is that it follows a particular order. It starts from the eastern quadrant, and it ends with the smell. You have to recollect in your mind all the processes, and see that since we are more concerned with man than anything else, the liver will have a more important place in the teaching. But it is necessary to be aware that they do not talk of the liver without talking of Jupiter or the odour.

Elisabeth Rochat: If you look at this translation you can see that there are two parts. The first part moves from the aspect of natural green to the cereal wheat. The second part begins with 'corresponding to the four seasons' and ends with the odour rancid.

In the first part the meaning is around the senses, the shapes, the aspect and appearance. It holds the sounds and shapes of the *qi* of earth. The senses are like a structure for all living beings in accordance with the *qi* of earth, *qi* which is transformed and changed by the presence of earth. In the first sentence there is an evocation of the space, the eastern quarter, which is a portion of space expressing a quality of *qi*. The second part is to do with the *qi* of heaven. We have the season spring, and the governor of heaven in time in the form of the planet Jupiter. I think this is the great division of space, the *qi* of earth and the *qi* of heaven. This description of the *qi* is just to expand on what the liver is, and what kind of *qi* is inside a human being.

SU WEN CHAPTER 5

The eastern quarter gives rise to wind,
wind gives rise to wood,
wood gives rise to acid,
acid gives rise to the liver,
the liver gives rise to muscular forces,
muscular forces give rise to the heart,
the liver masters the eye.

In heaven it is the mystery,
in man it is the dao,
on earth it is transformations.
Transformations give rise to the five tastes,
the dao gives rise to ability,
the deep mystery gives rise to the spirits.
The spirits, in heaven, are wind,
on earth, are wood.
Among the parts of the body it is the muscular forces,
among the zang,it is the liver,
among colours it is azure green,
among notes it is the note jue,
among noises it is the shout,
among movements that react to change it is to grasp,
among orifices it is the eye,
among tastes it is acid,
among the expressions of willpower it is anger.

Anger injures the liver, sadness prevails over anger.
Wind injures the muscular forces, dryness prevails over wind.
Acid injures the muscular forces, acrid prevails over acid.

SU WEN CHAPTER 5

Claude Larre: Chapter 5 seems to have more or less the same content as chapter 4, but this is never actually the case in a Chinese text. Due to the fact that four comes before five, four is more simple and five is more integrated, or integrating. Everything which has been said in chapter 4 is taken again here, but the perspective is not exactly the same, and we have to concentrate on the additional parts which make something new.

If we note here the place given to wind, we can understand that wind, which usually only has a pathological meaning, is also the essence of movement in the universe. We can see that it is a necessary link between east and wood. I will not make any further comment on this, but just give you the idea that chapter 5 is not simply a repetition of chapter 4.

Since 'muscular forces give rise to the heart' we find the connection between the liver and heart is made through the muscular forces (*jin* 筋). We understand that this force of life which expands so easily in any direction from the liver, now concentrates its power. Just as the winds concentrate their power in eight directions but come to a standstill because there is never any wind in the centre, so the heart is the silent governor protected by the liver. It is the central role of the heart to be the place where, being at a standstill, everything else is able to move by itself through the control of this motionless heart. It is so important to understand what true government is, and to see that true government is just the image of authentic life within an actual human being.

With the liver mastering the eye it is no longer a question of an opening or orifice, it is the relationship between the liver and the eye through this notion of mastering. Mastering gives more the impression of concentration.

In heaven it is the mystery
in man it is the dao
on earth it is transformations

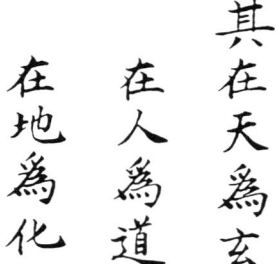

To understand the relationship between heaven and earth in man we have to understand that which we call the *dao* (道). The *dao* is proper to man, and a man following the *dao* is a saintly man. But what about the origin of the *dao* itself? Its origin is in the inscrutable mystery, so there is nothing to search out from heaven. Heaven is heaven, and you have to just say 'amen'! You have to stop, and if you do not, you are just a Westerner who wants to know the mystery of Chinese thinking, and there is no end to that process. Contemplation gets closer to the actual fact that life exists, and all descriptions of life lead you to that point where there is nothing to be seen, nothing to be heard, nothing to be touched. But on the surface of the earth we see the mystery of heaven multiplying itself in the diversity of the 10,000 beings, and not only separate beings but connected beings, and not stable beings but beings under constant change, all of which is registered in the Yi jing, the Book of Change.

Here we understand that there is a three-fold nature to what we want to know: the mystery, the *dao*, and the transformations. If you understand transformation you know life as a current, if you understand the *dao* you know how to conduct yourself, and if you accept the mystery you have to be reverent of what exists, whatever you may call it. This is the Chinese viewpoint, and not only Daoist because Confucius said just the same thing in his commentary on the Book of History, which was about the changes in the situation of his native place, the principality of Lu, and its relationships with other small kingdoms. The *dao* is not only proper to the Daoist. The *dao* is the rule you discover and practise, be you Daoist, Confucianist, Legalist, Mohist or Christian. They are all just ways of behaving between heaven and earth, and it is always the same heaven.

All this is found within a book of medicine. If you just treat people in order to relieve their pains, if you are not able to put them back on the right track in accord with the person they are and the situation they are in, then you are only doing half your work, and maybe you are wasting their time not to speak of your own.

Transformations give rise to the five tastes

化
生
五
味

The transformations of earth give rise to the five tastes, so the tastes are more important than the colours or sounds or the other things which go by the five systematic approaches to the perception of life. The tastes help build that which sustains life, and the stomach is the central part of posterior heaven. When an individual has been created you have to take care to maintain life or to restore it from a pathological state of illness.

The dao gives rise to ability

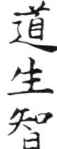

From there we come to what we call the mental sphere, which is not so distinctly presented in the Chinese text. They know that even if the spirits are more important than the *qi* or that the essences (*jing* 精) are more important than the *qi*, there is no spirit without a support for it, and there is no use for so much *qi* if it is not regulated by the *jing*. So it is up to us to make a distinction in the text, just to see that it runs smoothly from one statement to the other and not to insist on the differences too much.

When Elisabeth was talking recently of these different levels she did so because it was clear that something was pertaining to heaven and something was pertaining to earth, and that something was taken again to make an actual living being.

The distinction of mind, body and spirit is a sound distinction, but it is of no use in practice since the person there is just that one person. So if it helps you to make those distinctions then do so, but if it hampers your way of treating just keep them in your mind but do not insist on them too much, and do not try to find references to mind or references to spirit or references to body since they are always present in good books of medicine.

What is ability? In Chinese it means a knowing. The ideogram *zhi* (智) contains the image of an arrow going right to the centre of the target. Added to that is the ability to hit something centrally in any circumstance, whatever the target might be, and do it so deftly that nobody can see how you do it. That way of making a puncture, or assessing the condition of man, is the aim of the Chinese text, and is seen not only in the practice of acupuncture and medicine, but in every art and craft.

The deep mystery gives rise to the spirits

玄
生
神

What has been said of the *dao* is proper to man, and what is now said of the mystery is proper to heaven. The spirits in heaven are wind, so the wind which was not mentioned in chapter 4 now appears in the second part of chapter 5. This is important. It obliges the reader of the text to think about what might be the implication of wind and spirits. We know that the spirits come and go, and we know that the wind is coming and going. Therefore if the same motion is seen in wind and the spirits it is just because the wind and the spirits are more or less the same thing.

The spirits in heaven are wind
on earth are wood

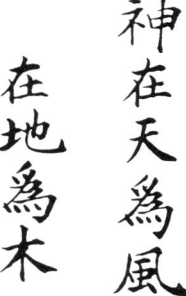

Elisabeth Rochat: Wind is only one of the expressions of the spirits in heaven, but it has a really special link with them because the wind is *yang qi*, like a messenger which brings us orders from heaven, and which can also take back something from earth. Wind is at the beginning of something because it is a first movement, the beginning of a movement, like an agitation or excitation. For this reason the wind is a special manifestation of the spirits, but only one manifestation of them. The spirits as a unity are an inscrutable mystery, but we can examine their effects.

Claude Larre: I just want to make a comment on what has been said from the so-called medical perspective, and what is seen in Chinese life, because we cannot separate Chinese structures of life from the study of medicine.

The spirits themselves on earth are also wood. This may seem strange, but there are many trees inhabited by spirits in the minds of Chinese folk. At the entrance to a village if there was an outstandingly beautiful tree it would be honoured because it was the residence of a spirit. Spirits were also in the earth, and the god of the soil in each village was honoured, and everything was thought to be more or less under his supervision.

So spirits are not only in heaven, they are everywhere, and in the case of the eastern quarter the spirits concerned are the spirits of wood, and wood is more visible than wind. Wind passes without you noticing, except if you see the leaves of the trees moving. In as much as there are spirits in heaven there must be spirits in wood, and you see them through the connection of heaven and earth.

Among the parts of the body
it is the muscular forces

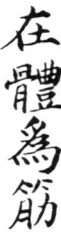

Among the zang it is the liver
among colours it is azure-green

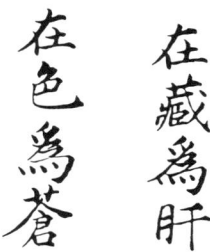

Claude Larre: This is not the same colour as in chapter 4 where it was *qing* (青). The azure green (*cang* 蒼) is the colour of heaven, as the granary (*cang* 倉) is a reservoir and a source, a spring for life and living.

Among notes it is the note jue
among noises it is the shout

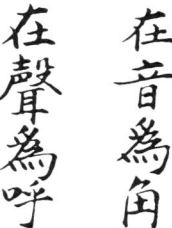

We have to understand that noises are sounds produced by man. This is a noise produced by some commotion, shouting. There is so much energy, and potential energy or condensed energy in the shouting that it is the proper movement of the column of air which is in the lungs and which goes up through the mouth. Therefore shouting is the true motion of the eastern quarter in so far as noises are concerned.

Elisabeth Rochat: The same ideogram has the meaning of shouting or expiring. It is the same because it is the same movement of breath as it goes out.

Claude Larre: Why do we have to choose between one meaning or another? Here it is because they are talking of noises, and a noise is more accurately described as shouting than expiring. But we also know that when a man is in a poor condition his breath makes more noise, it is not then just the expiry of the breath.

Elisabeth Rochat: The quality or quantity of expiration or inspiration is part of diagnosis.

Among movements that react to change
it is to grasp

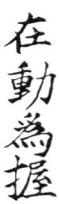

Claude Larre: We can all understand that I think. In Lao zi chapter 53 it is said that a young baby has a firm grasp. So the internal movement, the noise, and the external motion correspond one to another, shouting grasps the sound, and grasping an object is the equivalent of a shout.

Elisabeth Rochat: It is the same movement. The *qi* is in motion just as during the springtime.

Among orifices it is the eye
among tastes it is acid

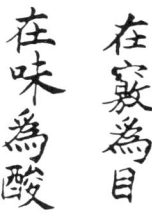

Among the expressions of willpower
it is anger

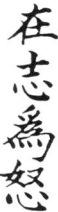

Claude Larre: The expression of the will (*zhi* 志) is connected with the power of life. If you want something with your will you are acting through the most essential part of your life power. So will and life power are identical at their root, and there is nothing intellectual which gets in the way in the

Chinese understanding. It is only in our own perception of will that we mix will and projection. The Chinese would say *yi* (意) if they wanted to talk of a projection because *yi* is concerned with the power of representing a proposal and having the power to act in order to realise what you have in your mind. In springtime anger is seen as the typical expression of the will. Anger is only one of the possible translations, and it is difficult because it sounds reproachful in our interpretation of language. It implies the same tension that you get when you draw a bow. In your mind, your willpower corresponds to anger. It is just tension.

Anger injures the liver
sadness prevails over anger

悲勝怒　怒傷肝

Wind injures the muscular forces
dryness prevails over wind

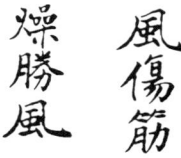

燥勝風　風傷筋

Acid injures the muscular forces
acrid prevails over acid

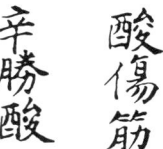

Elisabeth Rochat: The injury to the muscular forces from wind and acid is the same, like a spasm or cramp. They tense up the muscular force because the action of wind is an action of drying, but also of setting in motion. If this movement is too strong the result is a spasm. Acid normally has the effect of concentrating and contracting, so this is a good balance for the liver. It is also helpful in view of the liver's responsibility for keeping the blood. But if there is too much acid this action of collecting and strengthening is too strong, the muscular forces go into spasm and there is a blockage in the circulation of *qi.*

Question: Why is it said that marrow gives rise to the liver?

Elisabeth Rochat: This sentence actually appears in the section on the northern quadrant and the kidneys. In the same manner as the muscular forces give rise to the heart, the marrow gives rise to the liver. The text of chapter 5 here chooses marrow not bones because the basic substance of the liver is not found in *yang qi* or *yang* forces which are expressed in bones, but in *yin* matter and in the essences which are in the marrow. The marrow gives the power and strength to the bones. So this is an expression of the double nature of the kidneys. The essences of the kidneys give rise to the marrow and give rise to the blood, and the blood is stored by the liver as its fundamental function. All the other functions are effects.

Question: Could you enlarge on *zhi*, willpower, and its connection with emotion?

Elisabeth Rochat: Zhi (志) is not an emotion or a sentiment, it is a basic state from which all sentiment and emotion can take form. In the ideogram *zhi* (志) you see the heart in the lower part (心) and above is probably the image of a phallus. Something is erected on the earth in order to express life, and this is will, but without any consideration of emotion or sentiment. It is the foundation of the will for life, and with this connection between the kidneys and the heart, all emotion and feeling can take place through the heart. If the heart is void then there is a free circulation and permutation of all these emotions, which are just the same movements as the seasons or organs. But in the ideogram *zhi* there is a good basis and firm foundation.

If you look at Ling shu chapter 8 you can see that this *zhi* came after the good co-ordination of spirit, *shen* (神), *hun* (魂) and *po* (魄), after the heart is established as the centre, and after *yi* (意), the projecting of an idea which remains because it is good. So it is with the harmony with the whole of life in the individual that you have *zhi* (志).

Claude Larre: You make a decision to become an acupuncturist, but to carry it out it has to be shaped and well thought out. You have to know if you have enough time, what school you will apply to, what additional finances you need to support yourself. That is part of the construction of the scheme. Your idea is to become an acupuncturist, but this idea has to be built, and it has to rest somewhere in your will power.

Elisabeth Rochat: For the expression of life you need some expression of the movement of life and the emotions. You need both together in a good harmony to have balance in your mental life. If you have too much sadness you no longer have a spreading out, and this injures the liver. But if you have too much spreading out you need a little sadness to prevail over the anger.

Question: Can you say something about the significance of the placing of different parts of an ideogram?

Claude Larre: Usually the heart radical is seen on the left side or underneath. Sometimes, though rarely, it is in the middle of a character. On the left side it is more of an addition, it is to make the character more precise and to tell the reader that the character has something to do with the emotions and the heart. If the radical is underneath it gives the impression that everything rests on the heart. In this position the heart is understood as the basis for what is in the upper part. The position of the radical is important for meaning. If we talk of the earth radical, the earth is on the left or underneath, it is never on the right side. If it is the knife radical, it is always on the right side, and so on. So the combining is half convention, and half natural. For example, it is natural that a colour would be on the top.

The difficulty with Chinese characters is not only the position of radicals but the stroke order as well. In order to really understand that, you have to refer to Chinese lexicographers because they have taken years and years to establish how different parts combine.

Question: Could you say something about the ideogram for anger, *nu* (怒)?

Claude Larre: The lower part is the heart (心). The meaning is the impulse to begin something. For example, in Zhuang zi chapter 1 when the great fish in the ocean becomes a large bird-like creature and then leaves the water to move into the air; after a great effort and impulse it takes flight in the sky, and the effort is described by this ideogram *nu*. This is the effort to make life take off.

For the upper part I refer you to the Ricci Dictionary no. 3692 (*nu* 奴) which refers to slaves. Slaves are not educated people, they may be taken prisoner after a victorious war with the barbarians. They do not know the Chinese mind or culture, and their behaviour is always violent and impolite. Like French people compared to English people! If you have this feeling it ends in unrepressed conduct. You just do what you want, you express yourself with harsh words, you have no self-control, you are violent, and this violence is present in the spring and in anger.

Elisabeth Rochat: In the character for slave you have the characters for a woman on the left (女) and the right hand on the right. The woman was suppressed by the hand which created anger!

SU WEN CHAPTER 9

The liver is the trunk of extreme cessation
it is the residence of the hun.
Its flourishing aspect is in the nails,
its full power is in the muscular forces.
Its function is to produce blood and qi.
Its taste is acid,
its colour is azure blue.
It is the shao yang within the yang.
It has a free and easy communication
with the qi of spring.

Elisabeth Rochat: In this chapter the first characteristic of the liver is to be the 'trunk of extreme cessation' (*ba ji zhi ben* 罷 極 之 本). This expression is very odd because the other *zang* have a more noble definition of their charges. For example, the heart is the trunk of life and for all the changes through the spirits, and the lung is the trunk of *qi*.

Extreme cessation is the point where you have reached an extremity. It is the main beam in a building that holds everything together, the point where everything converges. At this place the liver assumes its function. It comes to a meeting point where it finishes everything and makes activity stop. We saw previously that the liver was in charge of the beginning of all activities, and this then seems contradictory.

But a cessation will also be the cessation of hibernation, and we have some texts such as the Huainan zi where this ideogram *ba* (罷) has the meaning of the cessation of sleeping, the cessation of inactivity and hibernation. This is the first point.

The second is that the ideogram *ba* (罷) is in two parts. The lower part is like a great brown bear, meaning that this implies the power and bravery of this kind of beast. This ideogram *neng* (能) means to be able to do something, to have the power to do something, the talent, the valour and the courage. The upper part is a net, and when all this power and strength is in a net, then you stop and you cease to exercise this power. There is a blockage and obstruction. It is the image of something entangled in a net so that it cannot express itself freely. If you put the heart radical underneath the character *neng*, you create another ideogram which is the expression of courage and bravery, the expression of internal value, *tai* (態). Every attitude which we show in our behaviour and gestures reveals the strength and power inside. When we talk of cessation in relation to the liver it is because one must economize and guard the force of life which is represented by the liver, to conserve, to manage and to regulate.

Question: I do not really follow why the liver is the trunk of extreme cessation. Do you mean it is because spring comes at the end of winter?

Elisabeth Rochat: The end of winter is the end of hibernation, but if you spoil your *qi* and your power you are unable to use your strength, and you are like a bear in a net. For this reason your muscular forces are completely exhausted and your *hun* are too, because this kind of exhaustion is on all levels. Your will is too exhausted to do anything. There is a relationship between the *qi* of the liver and gallbladder meridians and the brain and upper orifices. Therefore the liver is the trunk where all cessation of activity can occur. Zhuang zi chapter 15 says, 'The *hun* of a sage are never in this state of inactivity and ceasing.'

Question: Is this concept of the liver as the trunk of extreme cessation linked with *jue yin* (厥 陰), extreme *yin*?

Elisabeth Rochat: It is not the same ideogram. This ideogram for extreme in chapter 9 is *ji* (極), it is the point where everything meets, the ridgepole, the key position.

Claude Larre: If you take the lower part of the character *ba* (罷) there are three possibilities. You can leave it on its own as *neng*, meaning power or ability, associated with the *qi* of a bear. You know that different animals are different expressions of living forces and *qi* in the universe. In the northern abyss where there are big fish, the *qi* just waits like winter. But in the southern abyss there is a flying bird. That is the reason why you cast your Chinese horoscope in order to understand where your natural expression of *qi* is.

The point is that the bear has an exceptionally good position in all this since he is so powerful and strong when acting, yet so quiet when not moving. All this was observed by the Chinese.

If we put the net character on top of this, the net itself is an expression of capturing. Then we understand that the enormous *qi* which is represented by the bear is stopped.

The third possibility is to place the heart radical beneath the *neng* character so that it becomes the expression of the attitude which is the external manifestation of your inner self. This character is *tai* (態), and *tai* is an attitude, meaning that the *qi* is no longer seen as a bear, or the capturing of his energy, but just as a variegated expression of the *qi.*

At the beginning of Su wen chapter 1 there is much agitation surrounding the birth of Huangdi. The spirits are deeply moved and Huangdi appears, although they do not tell you whether it is through the motion of the spirits that he appears or if it is because of his appearance that they are moved! The classical Chinese text does not make a difference between the so-called cause and the so-called effect, it just states the thing as it appears. The second line comes to the second level where it is no longer a question of *shen* but a question of *jing* or *qi*. Here the text refers to Huangdi saying that he was able to express himself, and the characters used are *neng yan* (能 言). In ordinary language *neng* would mean to be able, but in an etymological context it means that you have enough *qi* to be able to do something. To be able does not refer to life as such, it is the qualities of your *qi* which make you able to write, to walk and so on.

Two years ago this character *ba* (罷) caused Elisabeth and I a lot of trouble. We were unable to understand why this extraordinary strength giving life, expanding in all directions, was also the trunk of cessation. We would say that on the contrary the liver is just the way life is expanding itself visibly. But here we have to say that it is impossible to be an expanding force if you are not also the force which keeps things under the ground in hibernation.

One part of Su wen chapter 1 talks about the numbers and cycles which rule a woman's and a man's life. For a woman it is seven, and seven periods of seven years which rule her life as far as fertility is concerned. It is not the age which is stated, it is the ascending phases, and the declining times, not just fertility, but the ability through fertility to use the supply of the surplus of life which is in her. For man it is eight, and eight periods of eight years making 64 years for the ability to bring life to a woman in order that through that woman he can perpetuate his own life by means of a child. Su wen chapter 1 says that in man at seven times eight years the *qi* of the liver declines, the muscular forces, *jin,* are no longer capable of moving.

The text here is so clear that it is not necessary to make too much comment, but I can just remind you that the muscular forces (*jin* 筋) are sometimes translated as muscles, sometimes as tendons. The muscle is not the flesh, the muscle is the flesh plus the ability to move. So tendons and muscles combine into one unit which is the basis for physical motion. When the *qi* originating from the liver declines, the external appearance of that decline is seen in the motion. It is no longer supple, full of strength and precise. Look at old people, they are hesitant, they fall easily, and so on. This is not just because the muscles and tendons are not strong enough, but because the liver is not giving enough *qi* to maintain the ability to move correctly in the muscle and tendons. The Chinese way is to observe external phenomena, whilst always keeping in mind that they are only the superficial appearance of a more profound state of life.

Elisabeth Rochat: We saw in Su wen chapter 1 the end of woman's fecundity and man's potency, and the implication of the liver *qi* in that, and this is precisely the beginning of the stopping of that movement.

We do not speak of the liver at the beginning of the power of man, but we know that the liver itself and its meridian has a function in the reproduction of life. It is just at the time when the *qi* is declining, in cessation, and is exhausting itself that we speak of it. So it is in the liver that the cessation of activity begins to be visible.

Claude Larre: We also need to think very carefully about the liver's assessment of circumstances and conception of plans, deciding when the armed forces have to move or stop and so on.

Elisabeth Rochat: 'It is the residence of the *hun*'. What are the *hun* (魂)? According to Zhuang zi the *hun* in a sage are never in a state of cessation. For this reason I think that there is in the idea of the *hun* a notion of activity which is not present in the *shen* (神). The *shen* which are kept by the heart are related to non-action. They are inexpressible, they cannot be analysed. The *shen* cannot even be reduced to analysis within *yinyang* because, being beyond them, they are what allow the deep, profound unity of each being. The *hun* follow the inspiration of the *shen*. For example, in Ling shu chapter 8 the definition of the *hun* is that which comes and goes conforming to, and modelling itself upon, the *shen*. They are therefore an expression of the activity inspired by the *shen*. As with the *shen*, their number is indefinite, it could be one, it could be many. It is never defined, and they are beyond all enumeration. But since the Han Dynasty there have always been three *hun*. They represent the activity which is directly inspired by the *shen* at the level of three, or on three levels, it is the same thing. Three is the number of *qi*, and the *hun* are on the side of activity, of *qi* and of *yang*. There is a unity in the *hun*, but it is a unity which is expressed in the unity of heaven, earth and man. For example in texts of internal alchemy the three *hun* are placed in the three cinnabar fields (*dan tian* 丹 田) in the head at the level of the brain, in the chest and just below the umbilicus, and the liver has a special relationship with each of these three areas.

Claude Larre: When talking of the three *hun* we usually have a tendency to try and separate out their different functions. But life itself is a unity and this unity is made when all parts of the body and the emanations of the three *hun* are working together. If we speak of 'mind' we are speaking of the *san hun* (三 魂), three *hun*, but if we want to talk of 'spirit' then it is no longer a question of the three *hun* but of the *hun* answering to a higher mystery, which is the *shen*. It is like being under the influence of some mysterious master who either does not speak or speaks only a few words, but who attracts your mind. They are so high above us that they express or they do not express, they are roaming free and we just try to adapt to them.

The distinction between the *shen* and the *hun* is that the *hun* are so connected with the body that each time you talk of them it is almost possible to differentiate the first from the second and the third from the first and second. They are on the level of life in the median, not the bones as such, and not the spirit, they are life itself which is on the move but which has to be referred to the highest level. The *shen* are free, and the *hun* adapt their movement to what they feel are the indications given them by the *shen*.

Elisabeth Rochat: The cataleptic state of the saintly man in meditation occurs when the *hun* have left the body for the mystic journey. He journeys with an aesthetic vision through the *hun*, whilst living a vegetative life. He has all the activities of life which ensure the maintenance of his body, but he is almost in suspended animation. He can no longer speak, he no longer sees, and he no longer has any means of expression. The function of the *hun* is thus explained by their absence. But through these journeys the *hun* puts the meditator in contact with the great and profound reality of life. This is possibly because of the close connection between the *hun* and the *shen* where the *hun* are ministers and auxiliaries for the *shen*. It is possible that through sleep and through dreams, where the liver and the *hun* play a fundamental role, that there is this same contact with the deep reality of your being. At death the *hun* are carried away by their natural movement of rising, expanding and diffusing. When there is no longer anything more to keep them together, to bring them back and hold them, then there is the dissociation of the *hun* and the *po* (魄), and that is death.

In China there is a traditional ceremony called *zhao hun* (招魂), the calling of the *hun*. When someone has just died they go to the roof of the house and call to the *hun* begging them to return to the body of the deceased. If they do not come back then the *po*, which have a movement of concentration and moving downwards, descend into the earth. The relatives and mourners try to make sure that the *po* stay in the body when it is in the tomb so that they do not come out and annoy the living. To do this they seal up all the exits of the body to trap the *po* inside. In funeral rites, when you are sure the *hun* are not going to come back, all the orifices of the body are plugged with rice or jade, depending on how rich you are. Then the body is placed inside a coffin, and that coffin is placed inside another coffin, and that is repeated several times. Finally all the coffins are put inside a tomb and it is sealed up.

To return to the *hun*, they have a movement of elevation and diffusion, and because of that there is a danger of dissipation and scattering. The *hun* need to be restrained, and they need the power of the *po* which are on the side of essence and structure, to fix them.

There is also another aspect to be considered which is that the *hun* express themselves or are expressed through the blood. In Ling shu chapter 8 it says that the blood is the residence of the *hun*. The liver stores the blood and therefore this red liquid which is so full of life, and which is linked to the heart and to the spirits of the heart, is also the vehicle for the activity of the *hun*. The *hun* need this mass of blood to fix them and give them something solid. Inversely, it is the lungs which store the *qi* and the *qi* is the residence of the *po*. The *po* are more on the side of essence and structure and of a movement which gathers and collects. This is the movement proper to *yin*. So the *hun* and the *po* are the *yang* and *yin* expression of the *shen*. The *shen* themselves are beyond what we can express through *yin* and *yang*, they are the radiance and illumination of life, as in *shen ming*. *Yin* and *yang* expressions of vitality are found at every level of life, and the *hun* and *po* are an archetype of *yin* and *yang* working in a human being. You must not lose sight of the fact that it is the penetration and crossing of the two which makes life.

Claude Larre: I would refer you to Lao zi chapter 10 where the first sentence is *zai ying po bao yi* (載 營 魄 抱 一). *Zai* means to maintain, *ying* is in place of *hun* and is all the activity of a superior type which has to rely on the *po*. You cannot be so angelic that you do not care for the servants who make life for you. You have to decide to maintain the *ying*, and if you are able to retain the unity of yourself, *bao yi*, then everything goes smoothly.

The interesting thing here is that it is the beginning of the part of the Daode jing where the conditions of life are stressed, and from chapter 10 onwards you see a difference in vocabulary. The text does not talk of *hun*. In medical texts you probably do find *hun* and *po*, and in books about rites and ceremonies you always find the three *hun*. The banner of Mawangdui is in itself a representation of what to do when the three *hun* go upwards and the seven *po* are left to care for the remains of the person. In other books different expressions are used, and if *hun* is not found then *ying* (營)

may be used. It is the activity of the *hun* which is alluded to. It means to nourish and infuse with life. The *po* do not make life come, they just serve life, and it is interesting to be able to make such a distinction between the more and the less noble activities in man, since the Chinese have always been taught to observe a social order.

Question: The *shen* are supposed to enter the foetus of the baby at the third month, when do the *hun* enter a human being? Is it only after birth?

Elisabeth Rochat: No, before birth. If the *shen* and the *hun* are really the powers which direct the movement necessary for life within the unity of the being which emerges from the void, then they must be there at the beginning of that being. There are non-medical texts which say that the *po* come first and then the *hun*, but this is just to say that the *jing* has to be there in order to produce the structure of a being, to give a code for the structure and to bring together all the constituents for a being. It is the blue-print or pattern. So if the *hun* express this movement of diffusion or circulation of life, and if they are the active expression of and for the *shen*, then they must necessarily be there at the moment when this power takes form.

There is no real before or after in the sense of time, there is only the mystery of a being, the mystery of life which is individual to a being and which can only be expressed through this double action of the *hun* and *po*. The right hand side of the characters for both *hun* and *po* is *gui* (鬼) which is a spirit of the earth. Therefore there is a differentiated expression in this being which takes life on this earth under heaven. If we look at it from the point of view of the *hun* we would say that they are for the expansion of life on the side of *yang*, and we would say that the *hun* are primordial. But if we look at the other side of the deep structure for life, at the essences which continually reconstitute your being, not only in your body but also in your spirit, then we would have to say that the *po* are primordial and come first. Birth is only a stage in the process of life, albeit a very important stage. There are different rites at different levels, but before birth and after birth are just different stages with different rituals.

Claude Larre: Why are we now talking of rites and leaving the field of anatomy and physiology? The point is that rites are the way to maintain order in the social body. Without rites it is impossible to make Chinese society function. Without something very close to rites it is impossible to make a human body or an individual live. Rites are the social aspect of the movement of life in an individual. Therefore on the question of what time the *hun* become active in a baby, the distinction might be very clear. If a woman is pregnant there is no child as such. There is a development of part of the woman which will, after birth, become another distinct individual. The child is part of the mother, and the *hun* and *po* of the mother are doing all the work, but they are slowly, indistinctly, forming what will become the *hun* and *po* of the child after birth. When you see that as a continuous process the question of what precise time does the *hun* knock on the door to enter the baby is nonsense. It is a koan. A koan is beyond sense in order to press the mind of the disciple to change his or her direction and try another approach to what is real. What appears as contradictory are just two sides of a question which will be solved on a higher level.

Question: You said that the *hun* gets its inspiration from the *shen*, so what gets out of balance? Are the *shen* to blame?

Claude Larre: No, the *shen* are always perfect.

Question: So how are the *shen* affected if the *hun* are not in order?

Claude Larre: The *shen* are just going elsewhere and doing other work. They do not even wait for the *hun* they are so independent and autonomous.

Elisabeth Rochat: If the *hun* are in disorder it is because there is a lack of communication between the *shen* and the *hun*. The *shen* cannot radiate their light sufficiently.

肝居膈下上着脊之九椎下。是經多血少氣其
合筋也其榮爪也主存魂開竅於目其系上絡
心肺下亦無竅○難經
曰肝重四觔四兩左三
葉右四葉凡七葉○滑
氏曰肝之爲臟其治在
左其臟在右脅右腎之
前並胃着脊目之第九椎

肝

The liver, from Lingshu suwen jieyao

PHYSIOLOGY AND FUNCTIONS OF THE LIVER

Elisabeth Rochat: We see from the texts of the Su wen and Ling shu that the liver is an essential organ in the human body, having the charge of general of the armed forces, which is in harmony with the nature of the liver, being very firm and correct, and being at the beginning of movement. There is a masculine force in the liver, and along with the heart it is referred to as a male organ because of this force which is directed to the expansion and diffusion of life. The spleen, lung and kidney are all called female.

It is the capacity for movement, decision, courage and firmness which characterizes the liver, and which is summed up in the sentence from Su wen chapter 8 about it being the general of the armed forces. But a general must not let himself be carried away. Through the inheritance of the *hun* it has the possibility of analysing and discerning, and of assessing situations and acting in accordance with them.

This facility is found in all the functions of the liver: in storing the blood, in the defence of the body, and its actions on the muscles.

The liver is described in the classics in an anatomical way which shows that the Chinese understood where the liver was in the body and what form it took. But we know that this anatomical description of the liver is only the visible manifestation of the liver in the material form of flesh and tissue. The function of the liver in traditional Chinese medicine is concerned with the profound movement which springs up and surges forth.

THE LIVER STORES THE BLOOD

Claude Larre: The Chinese character *cang* (藏) is not very easily translated into English. When we say 'store' it is the idea of keeping preciously, treasuring, or thesaurizing.

Question: How do we define that kind of storing?

Elisabeth Rochat: It is to keep actively, in such a way that by storing, all life may manifest. The effects of life can come from the storing. What we call the *zang* have the same ideogram (臟), and the *zang* are nothing more than five different ways of storing and treasuring the essences for the emission of *qi* and the continual structuring of life. You must never consider this storing like keeping something closed up in a box. It is to be full and to be steeped in the power of the *jing* and *qi*. This is to understand what each organ has to do for life and to have the means of doing it. For example, the liver has this movement of expansion and springing up which at the level of the body is seen in the muscles, or at the level of the mind in allowing the conception of plans.

Because the liver keeps the blood it allows the springing up of different effects, just as seeds germinating in the soil become flowers in springtime by means of the rising sap. This is all seen in the character for wood which is the element linked with the liver. An old Chinese explanation for this ideogram *mu* (木) is that you have the trunk planted vertically in the ground, you have the leaves and branches and you can see the roots beneath. That is to say it is only because there is a deep rooting that there can be a springing up towards heaven. Hence the first function of the liver is as the guardian and distributor of the blood. The liver stores but also releases it.

It says in Su wen chapter 10:

> *When a man is at rest the blood returns to the liver. The liver receives the blood and one can see.*

If the liver receives the right quantity of blood and sends it to the eye, the vision can be of good quality.

> *Feet receive blood and one can walk. The palms of the hands receive blood and one can grasp objects. The fingers receive blood and one can pick things up very carefully.*

At every stage of movement both the precision and the strength are reliant on the liver. It is the liver that has to release the right quantity of blood necessary for all muscular activity. It also has a nutritive role in that the blood itself has a general nutritive role for the *zangfu* (藏府), as well as for all layers of bodily structure, from the bones to the skin.

When a man is asleep or at rest with his limbs and muscles no longer working, and his orifices and sense organs closed and not functioning as they do when he is awake, then the blood returns to the liver and you have the activity of dreaming which comes about through the *hun* (魂).

If this function of the liver storing the blood is disturbed then the repercussions can appear in all activities of the body, for example in the quality of sight or in the muscular forces when a deficiency of liver blood gives rise to cramps and spasms. It can also affect joints and articulations, anything which involves bending and extending. This bending and straightening is the most fundamental aspect of the wood element. There can also be repercussions in a woman's menstruation, such as amenorrhoea, particularly if less blood is available. In certain classical texts the liver has also been called 'the sea of blood'. This brings it into direct relationship with *chong mai* (衝 脈), and we should remember that the third point on the liver meridian is called *tai chong* (太 衝), the powerful current, full of impetus and buoyant strength. This reminds us that *chong mai* (衝 脈) and *ren mai* (任 脈) are equally essential in the reproductive life of a woman, and certainly the liver is one of their heirs or assistants in this function of storing the blood.

THE FORMATION OF BLOOD

Elisabeth Rochat: The spleen has a double function in relation to the blood. Together with the stomach it extracts and works on the very concentrated, dense juices and liquids. By means of the pathway of *tai yin* (太 陰) there is a passage from the middle heater to the upper heater, and as these liquids are by then very pure, they can pass through the diaphragm. They are presented to the field of oxygenation in the lungs and then after that they go to the heart. There a radical change takes place. The blood becomes red because the heart has put its mark or stamp on the liquids which before were just very rich juices, but which then become blood. That is to say the blood is liquid which has the colour of fire and has the ability to bring life to the whole the heart that there is this radical change. References to the blood occur in chapters 18, 30 and 81.

The kidneys are also implicated in the blood because blood is a liquid which is more *yin* (陰) and linked with the *jing* (精). The kidneys have a certain function in regard to the blood which is because of their relationship to liquids via the quality of the *jing*.

Question: In some sources there is talk of marrow producing blood. Does the Nei jing elaborate on how marrow produces blood?

Elisabeth Rochat: Su wen chapter 5 says that marrow gives rise to the liver, and this is through the relationship with the essences, *jing* (精), of the kidneys. The *jing* of the kidneys is implicated in the constitution and in the quality of the blood because of their connection with the original or innate constitution of the being. It is the *jing* of the kidneys which makes up the marrow. The kidney and liver have this relationship through the *sheng* (生) cycle, so the easiest way of summing all this up is to say that the marrow gives rise to the liver. But there are no classical Chinese texts which directly link the marrow and the blood.

Question: Do the kidneys have a role in the quantity of blood as well?

Elisabeth Rochat: Every organ has some effect on the quantity of blood, each according to its different nature. If the stomach and spleen do not have anything to eat then there will not be the quantity of blood, or it will be impoverished. There is never just one organ responsible for one area of life, you cannot say that just one organ is responsible for the blood. For each organic reality there is a crossing of all five movements that make life.

THE LIVER AS MASTER OF
FREE FLOW AND CIRCULATION

Elisabeth Rochat: Another function of the liver is that of making free circulation and flow, allowing everything to penetrate easily and spread everywhere. We can recognise the power of spring in this, and the power of the beginning which is in *shao yang* (少 陽) to remove all obstacles and create free movement. This circulation is made through spreading and elevation, which is what we saw previously in regard to the spring in Su wen chapter 2. This is taken up again in chapter 18 where each of the five *zang* is discussed in the context of its own movement in relation to the storing of what is real and authentic, of what is most deep in a being and which makes them an individual. The movement of the liver is that of diffusion, which is expressed particularly through the muscles, but also through all the connective tissues in the body, all the fascia.

So the great tendency of the *qi* of the liver is to spread out everywhere, ensuring that good circulation is created everywhere because the first impulse is given with sufficient strength. But this has to be differentiated from the function of the heart which has mastery over all the life-giving network, the *mai* (脈).

It should also be contrasted with the function of the lungs which are involved with the rhythm that is given to this circulation. You have to make a very close connection between the function of the liver spreading out and springing up, and the function of ascending and descending in the body which is linked with all the *zang* and *fu*. For example, the lungs make the *qi* and liquids descend, while the bladder and kidneys act as a foundation for the rising up of *qi* and *jing*. Obviously the central mechanism of the stomach and spleen directs elevation and descent, and is itself kept in balance by the wood element and the liver's movement of free circulation.

THE LIVER AND THE EMOTIONS

Elisabeth Rochat: The loss of the liver's function of making free flow has repercussions on the circulation of *qi*, particularly on the movement of raising and lowering. But one of the greatest manifestations of this function in the body is free circulation in regard to the emotions. The ideogram for emotion, *qing* (情), is composed of two parts, the heart on the left side and *qing* (青), the natural green colour, on the right. This indicates that the same liveliness and vivacity which manifest in springtime and in the east, when related to the realm of the heart give us the ideogram we translate as emotion. It is because of this that the liver is given a great place in the governing of the emotions. What is important about emotions is not whether they exist or not, there are always different movements which we call fear or anger or whatever, but whether they are in balance and harmony, and whether they are in free circulation. Nothing should block them. If an emotion is blocked then the *qi* which forms the emotion will become pathological. Emotions are nothing more than the expression of *qi*, and when that is obstructed it will give rise to feelings which are not normal.

This particular responsibility of the liver for the emotions also comes from the fact that the liver stores the *hun*, the spirits which are closest to the *shen*, and therefore linked with the higher aspects of the mental and emotional sphere.

In addition to all this each *zang* has a particular expression in the realm of the emotions by which the *qi* that constitutes a *zang* also constitutes the same movement in the realm of emotions. For the liver its quality of springing up and spreading out gives it an impetuosity which when it becomes pathological is excessive anger. Anger takes someone over and carries the *qi* upwards in the body, it makes you lose control of yourself. All this has repercussions on the *hun* and the storage of blood. When anger is very strong and the fire within the anger is very powerful, then the blood and all its constituents are impoverished. There is a drying up of the blood and at that time the *hun* no longer have a proper residence and they become dissipated.

There is a warning given in many classical texts that you have to be careful if you are nourishing or relaxing the liver that you do not release anger. Certain commentators go even further than this and say it is better to tonify the kidneys, which will have a secondary effect of tonifying the liver, rather than tonifying the liver directly.

On the other hand states which we might think are physical can also have an effect on the emotions. For example, if there is too much richness in the constituents that form the blood then this can bring about a tendency to anger. If there is an emptiness in the blood, then there will be an emptiness in the liver and gallbladder and there will be a tendency to be fearful. If there is an emptiness in the *qi* of the liver then there is an emptiness in the *qi* which gives the ability to push outward and forward in life. The result is that there is a kind of recoiling which takes the form of fear. So the harmony between the blood and *qi*, between the *yin* and *yang* within the liver is necessary to ensure the free circulation of the *qi* which forms the emotions.

Two different emotions affect the liver most, when someone is too excited or is very depressed. When the liver *qi* can no longer ensure this free circulation it is obstructed or knotted. It does not flow smoothly and the person becomes oppressed and joyless, suspicious of others and mistrustful. If you want to put that into a five element framework it is the lung *qi* and its sadness which submerges the emotion of the liver.

Claude Larre: This feeling of sadness is proper to autumn. There is less light in the sky, your summer vacation is behind you, and work is starting again. All that gives some kind of distress or oppression, and might be able to block that flux of energy and vitality and joy which is more proper for the liver.

Elisabeth Rochat: On the other hand the thought and reflection which are linked to the earth element can come across the reverse *ke* cycle and attack the liver. If the liver no longer has the ability to conceive of things and to transform thoughts and reflections into plans, then you are just left going round and round with the same thoughts. At the same time you can also observe swellings, blockages and obstructions in the region of the ribs and thorax.

body because it is penetrated by the power of the *shen*.

Therefore the spleen has the function of elaborating the very rich liquids which form the basis of the composition of blood. The heart puts its stamp on these liquids, and the colour red is the seal showing the presence of the spirits. It is through its pulse and all the *mai* (脈), the life-giving network of vital animation, that the heart directs and maintains the free circulation for life. The spleen's relation to the blood lies in maintaining its form and keeping it in place. For example, haemorrhage and extravasation are symptoms coming from the spleen. This is different from having too much blood, it is rather that the blood is no longer in its proper place.

Question: I believe there is a quote from a chapter of the Ling shu which says that the blood is already formed in the stomach. Is that not right, that the remains of the food turn red?

Elisabeth Rochat: The Ling shu does not say that the blood is formed in the stomach. There is an elaboration of the juices which serve as the basis for blood in the middle heater, but blood is only called *xue* (血) when it is at the level of the lungs and heart. The stomach is the origin of blood because it provides the material from which it is composed, but blood is not made in the stomach. The red colour comes from the heart, and it is only when it reaches

When the blockage of the *qi* becomes very serious you can fall into a very profound depression, with constant weeping. The blockage which you can see in the emotions is also seen in the circulation of *qi* and blood, and has physical repercussions, such as dysmenorrhoea in a woman, for example.

The reverse case is over excitement, when the *qi* of the liver gets out of control and you have signs of agitation and disturbance. The person becomes anxious and agitated, is easily angered, and this can lead to insomnia and to lots of dreams if there is an effect on the *hun*. Being carried away like this can give trouble in the region of head, for example blurred vision and vertigo, or noises in the ears which can become so bad that they can cause deafness. Being carried away like this the fire of the liver rises up and affects the head and brain, and the eye and ear are implicated. The liver meridian passes over the head and through the brain to *du mai* 20 (*bai hui* 百 會) and the gallbladder meridian also goes over the head.

BLOOD CIRCULATION

Elisabeth Rochat: Blood and *qi* are inseparable. The image which is often given in Chinese is that of a person and their shadow. When the *qi* circulates the blood circulates, and when the *qi* is blocked the blood is blocked. When the *qi* of the liver is attacked the blood of the liver is attacked and if the *qi* of the liver is injured then it will affect the blood and vice versa. So a defective circulation of liver *qi* will have repercussions on the liver's function of storing the blood in two different ways. First, if there is a blockage and the *qi* cannot circulate freely then neither can the blood, and this can lead to sharp pains in the thorax and sides or to dysmenorrhoea. It can go further to produce stagnation and extravasation, with blood clots, tangible masses or amenorrhoea.

On the other hand if there is too much animation then the blood will be carried away and carried upwards because of the upward movement of the liver *qi*. Then the face and eyes become red, and in serious cases there can be bleeding from the nose or vomiting of blood.

There can also be a third situation which is a complete disorder in the circulation of the liver *qi* - the blood is no longer kept in its place of reserve, which can manifest in all kinds of haemorrhages. When you have this situation of obstruction in the free flow of the liver, heat is produced which can evolve into fire. This heat and fire seek to move and this can be one of the causes of what is called internal wind.

DIGESTION AND ABSORPTION

Elisabeth Rochat: The function of the liver to allow free circulation is also an important aid to digestion and absorption. The movement of the liver in making things flow is very helpful for the stomach and spleen in their role of ascending and descending. It also helps the gallbladder with the emission of bile. In fact the free circulation of *qi* under the impulse from the liver is one of the essential conditions for normal digestion and assimilation. If this does not happen you can have disturbance in the raising and lowering function of the stomach and spleen, such as belching and eructations, because the stomach *qi* is not lowered properly, or swelling of the abdomen because the spleen *qi* is not raised properly.

RELATIONSHIP WITH THE TRIPLE HEATER

Elisabeth Rochat: As well as the links between the liver and the middle heater, this function of the liver to make free circulation and flow affects all three heaters since it is a question of the good regulation of all the mechanisms of *qi*. The circulation of *qi* also has an effect on the circulation of liquids. For example, you could have a case of oedema or blockage by water which will come under the general framework of the triple heater, but where you might have to look to the liver for the cause. Here again we find the action of *shao yang* (少 陽) which unites the gallbladder and triple heater and has this function of pushing to the front and making everything circulate everywhere.

The circulation of everything which makes for free flow must occur with great ease and fluidity. It is for this reason that we can say that in its deepest nature the liver is *yin* while all the effects that spring from it have a *yang* nature. When there is complete harmony in the liver there will be an invigoration of the *qi* which with the firm basis of the *jing* and blood springs up and spreads throughout the whole organism to bring life to every element in the body.

RIGHT AND LEFT

Elisabeth Rochat: In Su wen chapter 52 it is said that the liver gives life by the left. In other texts it says that its treatment is by the left. We know that the liver is situated on the right hand side in the *yin* part of the body, but it is always related to the left side because its movement always goes towards the left. In other words from the basis of the *yin* the effect will be *yang*. This will be understood by those who do *tai qi quan* (太 極 拳). When you want to make a movement that goes towards the right you never do it directly, it is always necessary to begin with a movement of leaning towards the left, and then you can go towards the right with all the power of that movement.

In certain contexts it is said that the right hand side of the body is *yin* in relation to the left. The venous system goes on the right side and the arterial system goes in on the left. The heart which moves is more on the left side while the liver which stores is more on the right side. If you want to bring out a gesture, a movement or an effect, it must always be initiated on the opposite side. The liver stores the blood by regulating its quantity. It is therefore apparently located in the *yin* on the right side. All the movements that come from it are initiated on the right but have their effect on the left. So when you want to treat the liver for anything connected with its relationship with the *qi* then you might prefer to treat on the left side. On the other hand, the left (when one is facing south) is the place of the rising sun, opposed to the right, the west, the place of the setting sun. So, the left symbolises the rising movement and the right the descending one.

Claude Larre: It is more a question of the movement between two things than a question of right and left. This is not the case in western books of medicine where first a description is given to tell you where it is, and then later it is put in motion and the physiology starts. This is the distinction made by western medicine between anatomy and physiology which is a separation characterizing that sort of medicine.

The Chinese observe phenomena, and what they observe is always changing, so they are interested in the movement. They are interested in what is in the middle, in the void, because it is in that void that movement is possible.

THE MUSCULAR FORCES

Elisabeth Rochat: A more tangible and visible expression of the *qi* of the liver is in the muscular force (*jin* 筋), all the system of connections between the flesh and bones. It is this which allows articulations to move and enables precise movements to be made. It is also its strength which allows to you pick up objects with precision.

There is something called *zong jin* (宗 筋) which is translated as ancestral muscle. It means that all the muscles have a principle of direction and co-ordination and a gathering together in the same way that the ancestor gathers together the whole family. All the members of a family can be united in the same state of mind if the ancestor has a strong personality. The *zong jin* is located in the perineum and commands everything which is connected with the muscular forces in the body. The region of the perineum is important because it is there that the movement which exemplifies vital force is found, a man's erection. An erection has the movement of straightening and pushing upwards which is precisely the movement of life. The erection is only one aspect of reproduction, and only one aspect of everything which is concerned with muscular forces, but it is a very good correspondence and representation.

According to Su wen chapter 44 *zong jin* has mastery over bones which are joined to one another, which is one way of referring to the vertebral column. The bones have to be well connected to function properly with the possibility of movement, particularly bending and straightening in the way that wood does. The spine also permits all other movements in the body.

The supply of *qi* and blood are equally necessary for the good functioning of the muscles. The mastery of the liver over the muscular forces is connected with its functions of allowing free flow of *qi* and storing the blood, because it is through the nutritive power of blood that all movements and activities are possible. Movements which are too violent and impetuous will exhaust this function of the liver, as can be seen in Su wen chapters 4 and 9. When the liver no longer assumes its command over the muscular forces, especially if it is linked to an insufficiency of blood in the liver, the blood is no longer nourishing the muscles and you see symptoms such as trembling, often in hands and feet, leading in extreme cases to paralysis of the limbs and greater and greater difficulty in using the joints. Bending and straightening are no longer possible. If heat is added to this state it damages the body fluids and dries them up, further diminishing the quality of the blood. There could then be more violent symptoms such as spasms or cramps, episthotonos when the back is bent over or trismus, lockjaw. All these symptoms are also linked to liver wind. Liver wind brings a certain violence and speed to these symptoms.

THE NAILS

Elisabeth Rochat: What are nails? Muscles have the same *qi* as the *qi* of the liver, but are expressed inside the body. You cannot see them, but you feel them and you can see their effects. As this *qi* pushes further and further towards the exterior it forms what we call the nails. These are visible on the outside, and for this reason Su wen chapter 9 says 'its flourishing aspect is in the nails'. It is the same *qi* that creates the liver, is expressed in the muscles, and which finishes this movement of pushing to the exterior by forming nails. It is because of this that you can form conclusions about the state of the liver by looking at the nails. When the liver is working well the nails will be well nourished by the flow of blood and shining with health. They will be firm but also supple. Conversely when the liver is not in a good state of health the nails will be thin and soft. Soft is not the same as supple. They will be very brittle and easily split. They will have a fibrous aspect and be ridged.

THE EYES

Elisabeth Rochat: We have seen that the liver opens its orifice at the eye, so the power of its *qi* comes out there. This allows you to see into the distance. It is the same expression of the *qi* as in its ability to spring up with vitality. Good vision has its root in the irrigation and nutrition of the blood and *qi* of the liver, and it is their harmony which allows us to distinguish the five colours. It says in Ling shu chapter 17 'you can correctly grasp all the aspects presented on the outside of things', which is what we saw previously in regard to the aspect (*se* 色) and the idea of grasping the exterior aspect of beings. So anomalies in the functioning of the liver will have repercussions in the eye and in vision. Insufficiency of the *yin* of the liver or the blood of the liver will make the eyes dry, blur the sight or cause night blindness. With wind and heat in the liver you have blurred vision and vertigo or strabismus.

THE HEAVENLY STEMS

Question: Can you please explain a little about the characters for *jia* (甲) and *yi* (乙) which are the first two heavenly stems and which are connected with the liver and gallbladder?

Elisabeth Rochat: In the Yue ling, 'Commandments for each

Month', which is part of the Book of Rites, we find it said that the names most suitable to the days of spring are *jia yi* (甲 乙). That is to say there is in these names something that is very similar to the movement of spring.

Jia (甲) is the idea of a very hard tree bark, of scale and of armour. The traditional Chinese etymology for this ideogram is the image of a helmet on the head of a big man. It is the idea of something that envelops and at the same time protects, like a tortoise shell. It also has the meaning of the claws of a bird, its talons. It is the sense of gripping something very tightly in order that something can come out of it, there is very great strength in that protection.

In the second character *yi* (乙) there is the idea of the seed of a plant which makes an effort to come out from the earth, piercing the surface. In this ideogram there is a notion of effort and impulse. So the meaning of both these ideograms is to burst out, open up, to germinate, spread out and diffuse. There is very great strength which is turned towards protection, but which is also capable of piercing through this protection in order to spring up.

Claude Larre: In addition to that we have to understand the relationship between *jia* and *yi*. *Jia yi* is the movement of life as it bursts out from the chaos.

Elisabeth Rochat: There is a classical text called the Jiayi jing which is the first attempt at an ordered classification of all the data given in the Nei jing. Here the meaning is 'The ABC of Acupuncture and Moxibustion'. *Jia, yi* and the other heavenly stems are often used in this way, to express all kinds of series, such as a, b, c, one, two, three etc.

In the movement manifested by *jia yi* there is all the strength of the wind which brings the thawing after winter. There is the idea of the animals which were hibernating just beginning to move and the fish which were at the bottom of the river coming back up to the surface. It is the moment of heaven and earth coming together again after the separation of winter. Once again the *qi* of heaven can descend and the *qi* of earth can ascend.

JUE YIN

Elisabeth Rochat: It is through all this that we can understand what *jue yin* (厥 陰) is. In the ideogram *jue* (厥) there is a double idea. On the left of the character there is the idea of vegetation which is pushing up (Wieger Lesson 102D) with the horizontal stroke indicating resistance and an obstacle to overcome. If you combine this with the radical for walking you have the ideogram *ni* (逆) meaning countercurrent. The right part of the character gives the idea of respiration or breathing which is blocked, and therefore contains the idea of suffocation. So in *jue* there is a sense of an obstacle to cross or a current which is inverted.

Related to *yin*, it is as if the *yin* has come to the end of itself and has come to the beginning of *yang*. It is just like when you have gone right through the night and you are at the moment when dawn is about to break, or when in winter the water is frozen and earth is hard, and they no longer seem to receive the warmth of the sun, then the opposite movement seems to begin at that point. In the depths of this situation which is winter, there is the seed which is capable of continuing its movement and breaking out and letting the circulation flow freely. So we can see quite well how *jue yin* is very suitable for the liver and how it is rooted in water, in the kidneys and winter, which represent the basis from which the impulse can be started.

CAUSES OF DISEASE IN THE LIVER

WIND

Elisabeth Rochat: One of the principle causes of disease from the exterior is wind. Wind breaks up the connection between the *ying qi* (營 氣) and the *wei qi* (衛 氣) which then increases agitation and disturbs the natural movement of the liver. Wind by its nature makes things rise, and will therefore provoke the functions of the liver and create something which goes too far. It induces an over-reaching in the rising and circulating movements which are natural to the liver.

Wind is amongst the perverse evils, and the one that can combine most easily with the others. It has a *yang* nature and can combine with fire or heat, both of which have a similar nature to wind itself. In this case there will be a movement of agitation and an exaggerated rising upwards. One of the greatest repercussions is obviously in the realm of *yin*, blood and body fluids. Wind can also combine with cold or with damp, and then it produces blockage and obstruction, cold being that which freezes and hinders free circulation. In that case there will be both agitation and disturbance from the wind and also obstructions preventing free circulation.

Wind can also combine with dryness, and in this instance there are two possibilities. With a warm nature it has a destructive effect on the interstitial fluids and all the body liquids and there will be a kind of vapour which evaporates and diffuses. In this case we find symptoms of elevation, circulation, movement, impediment and impoverishment of the *jin ye* (津 液), the bodily fluids. When dryness is linked with cold there will be symptoms such as blockage in the circulation and poor distribution of fluids. These symptoms are very difficult to distinguish because they are very intricate, but there are symptoms that can be differentiated.

EMOTIONS

Elisabeth Rochat: We have seen that the seven emotions injure the liver, and in particular anger which makes the *qi* rise upwards. Anger is something that excites the movement of the liver and has many repercussions. It can cause swellings in the thorax or affect the stomach and spleen. For example, in Su wen chapter 39 it says that when there is anger the *qi* reverses its normal flow and runs countercurrent. When this is very strong and intense it can produce vomiting of blood or diarrhoea with undigested food. If anger introduces complete disorder and reverses the normal storage of the blood by the liver some texts indicate that there is a strong possibility of uterine haemorrhage.

Anger can come from an external situation or from a more internal cause. Other emotions can also injure the liver such as fear, which makes the *qi* descend preventing its circulation. The *jing* turns in on itself. If there is a break between the different stages within the three heaters, then we can understand how the functions of the liver, which are to make things circulate and spread out, and to make things rise, get into difficulty since they are contradicted by this emotion of fear which draws downwards and blocks below. We can also see that the kidneys are injured by fear, so it is only with difficulty that they can serve as a basis and foundation for the liver and the springing up of life.

If there is the emotion of grief or oppression (*you* 憂) one no longer feels full of joy and liveliness. One is turned in on oneself without the possibility of opening up. The character shows the heart in the middle being squeezed in a vice between the top and bottom parts. The movement of this emotion is therefore the opposite to the natural movement of the liver in circulating and spreading out. If this state of oppression lasts a long time then there will be a break in the relationship between the liver and the middle heater.

For this reason, the person would gradually lose the desire to eat or drink, and there could be swelling in the sides and thoracic regions.

There is another emotion which can injure the liver, and that is fright (*jing* 驚) which is usually linked to the heart and to *xin bao luo* (心 包 絡). *Xin bao luo* (or pericardium) is also linked to the liver via *jue yin* (厥 陰). Fright may cause a loss of communication with the heart, a disorder in the functioning of the heart as master and in the communication that it has to have with all the other *zang* to give them the light of the *shen* (神). This affects the *hun* (魂) of the liver and can cause bursts of rage, insomnia, and disordered dreams. The liver loses its function of being able to conceive plans and assess circumstances, and there is disorder in the *shen*. Here you can see quite clearly the relationship of *jue yin* between the liver and *xin bao luo*. You can also see the communication of the liver with the eye and brain.

Claude Larre: We understand that the rest period during the night is the time for the *hun* to communicate with the heart, and this generates a state of stability and clarity, even if there are dreams during that time. In the morning when you come back to your senses the basis for the use of those senses relies on the rest of the night. The new energy which comes to life each morning is only possible because the night has been full of communication between the *hun* and the heart.

ALCOHOL

Elisabeth Rochat: Alcohol is humid, damp and also warm. It disturbs the realm of consciousness and the emotions, and can make your head spin and make you vomit. We find these symptoms in the actions of the liver and in the effects of the liver on the spleen. In the Nei jing it is said two or three times that alcohol is referred to in relationship to the liver and gallbladder.

SEXUAL EXCESS

Elisabeth Rochat: Sexual excess can also injure the liver, because although the attack is made directly on the kidneys, the deterioration in the kidneys will be felt by the liver. The liver loses that which nourishes it, and if the *jing* of the kidneys deteriorates and the liver blood is no longer sufficient or of good enough quality to retain the impulse of the liver to go upwards, then this is called an excess of liver *yang* caused by an emptiness. In this case we find symptoms such as hypertension, with its origin in kidney emptiness.

LIVER FUNCTIONS AND RELATED SYMPTOMATOLOGY

PUSHING AND SURGING UPWARD
(sheng fa 升 發)

Elisabeth Rochat: When this is in excess then the *qi* and blood will be brought up to the top of the body as if by a current of great strength. Then the parts of the body which will be affected are at the top, in the region of the head, and in the middle. This will often indicate that wind is involved. You can have pains in the head, blurred vision, and sometimes swelling. In the middle region you can have pains in the thorax and sides. If this excessive rising up manages to injure the descending function proper to the stomach then you have symptoms such as vomiting. If in addition there is such a great strength in this pushing upward that it makes the liver lose its function of storing the blood then there will be blood in the vomit or spitting of blood.

If, on the other hand, this function is deficient there will be difficulties in the *qi* and blood rising and diffusing. In that case there will be symptoms indicating the lack of supply of *qi* and blood to the head, such as dizziness on getting up from lying or sitting, and pains in the head which are relieved by pressure. This deficiency can also cause swellings which are intermittent.

FREE CIRCULATION AND FLOW
(*shu xie* 疏 泄)

Elisabeth Rochat: When this aspect is in excess symptoms will be more visible in the middle and lower parts of the body. There may be illnesses such as *xiao ke* (消 渴), which is often translated as diabetes, where the principal symptoms are great thirst and frequent urination. There can be sudden diarrhoea with a pressure in the lower abdomen, and some kind of tenesmus. For women, since the blood is no longer stored because of too much circulation and flow, the quantity of blood during a period will be abundant, and the period can even come too early. In serious cases this can lead to a uterine haemorrhage.

When this function of free circulation and flow is deficient then you can have a pain in the thorax with a sensation of oppression within all the cavities of the middle region due to lack of circulation. The person may try to regain the circulation by sighing and deep breathing. In the lower part

nere can be anuria, and some kinds of blockage
⸴ pains in the lower leg. In gynaecology it is the
ıcture to the one for excess circulation: the period
comes ıⲖte and there is a tendency for there to be less
blood. There can also be clots, lumps and obstructions
which cause pain.

MOTION AND SHAKING
(dong yao 動 猺)

Elisabeth Rochat: When this is too strong the attacks will be
on the *jin mai* (筋 脈), the vital life-giving network which
brings the *qi*, blood, nourishment and irrigation to all the
tendons and ligaments, and which permits movement of
the joints. The liver governs all this movement, and should
keep it within limits, but when there is too great a force
moving through the *jin mai* then the strength of this movement
in the form of wind will cause disordered and abnormal
movements. In this situation you can have all kinds of
nervous ticks and twitches. You see people who are always
shaking or moving their heads, who have Bell's Palsy or
facial spasms. There can be blurred vision as well. These
are all symptoms that arise from disturbance in the *jin mai.*

When this function of motion and shaking is deficient then
you have muscular contractions because the supply of

nutrition through the *jin mai* is insufficient. Because of the absence of this irrigation you have cramps, spasms and muscular contractions which can reach the point of paralysis if the lack of nutrition lasts a long time. You could also have Bell's Palsy from deficiency because in this case a secondary sort of wind could arise from the emptiness of body fluids. If this situation persists then a *yin* deficiency can occur leading to a destruction of the person's *shen* (神) due to the resulting heat. It destroys the *shen* and the *hun* (魂) and the relationship between them, so there is no longer any peace. In very serious cases this can reach a point of unconsciousness, or mental disturbance where people no longer know what they are doing or saying. The direction in the mental sphere which should be given by the liver and gallbladder is no longer there.

Whether there is excess or deficiency in motion and shaking, both will finally lead to a situation of internal wind and consequent agitation and disturbance. When it is too strong the action is more direct, and there are different kinds of ticks and twitches, with the agitation seen on the outside quite visibly, particularly at the top of the body on the head. When it is too deficient the circulation and irrigation of the *jin mai* is insufficient. From this there is an attack on the function of the muscular forces because nutrition is lacking. This emptiness leads to a secondary effect like the wind which produces movements of shaking in the hands, or heat which disturbs the spirits and speech. Since it springs from a weakness in the liver this then prevents the good functioning of the *hun*, and the good analysis of circumstances and correct behaviour.

BLURRED VISION

Elisabeth Rochat: In vertigo with blurred vision there can be two different causes which are linked to the liver. First it can be a symptom of the fullness of the *yang* of the liver, where the liver wind rises upward causing trouble in the vision. In this case you have a head which turns and there may even be swellings in the head area and a buzzing in the ears which is like the noise made by the sea's tide. At the same time when you examine the urine you will see that it is yellow, indicating the presence of heat. The eyes will be red and the mouth will have a bitter taste, while the tongue will be red with a yellow coating. There may be agitation with a tendency to anger.

The second cause of blurred vision is emptiness of the blood of the liver. In this case you have the same vertigo and dizziness, and also perhaps the swelling, but the buzzing in the ears is like the song of crickets, with variations in the intensity. At the same time you can have swellings in the sides and thorax.

HEADACHES

Elisabeth Rochat: When headaches are caused by an interior attack on the liver they will begin slowly and intermittently. There are several categories within this division, for example when the *qi* of the liver or gallbladder meridian is blocked there will be headaches which are mostly one-sided or in the region just above the eyebrows. In this instance you can still sometimes observe swelling in the thorax and sides.

If the headaches are caused by the liver *yang* rising too strongly, for example if the supply of liquids to the liver is insufficient, then you will have vertigo and blurred vision along with a buzzing in the ears accompanying this type of headache. If it is not just the *yang* of the liver which rises due to the fire, this is one stage worse, and the difference is that the fire disturbs what is pure and makes the body fluids unclear. For example, in the region of the middle heater there will be the formation of phlegm. For this reason you have uneasiness and discomfort in the heart region. You also have symptoms of fire such as red eyes, bitterness in the mouth, a tendency to anger and yellow urine. There will not just be headaches but disturbance of the upper orifices and of the body fluids which should irrigate and nourish them.

With headaches which come from cold entering the *jue yin* (厥 陰) you have a pain at the vertex of the head, the highest point that the meridian of *jue yin* reaches in the region of *du mai* 20 (*bai hui* 白 會). There are also symptoms of cold present, such as clear vomit or saliva. The Chinese classics describe the pulse when there is cold in the *jue yin* as lax or without tension. There will also be buzzing in the ears.

When tinnitus is a symptom of fullness, for example when liver fire is the cause, there is a brutality about it, and there is a sudden starting in the sound like a tide. On the other hand when buzzing in the ears is caused by emptiness due to insufficiency of kidney *yin* which is therefore unable to correctly nourish the liver, there is a secondary phenomenon of disharmony between the *yang* of the liver and the blood of the liver. The *yang* rises and causes the buzzing in the ears, and the blood and essences of the liver are unable to irrigate the brain and inner ear. The onset of this will be slower, and you have an intermittent noise described as being like cicadas.

MENSTRUATION

Elisabeth Rochat: The liver stores the blood. Therefore when the liver blood is deficient the quantity of blood in the period diminishes. It is also said that the colour of the blood changes and becomes paler. In serious cases this can lead to amenorrhoea.

A second point is that the liver commands the circulation and free flow, and it is this function which makes the storing of blood all the more important. The liver therefore controls both the storing and the giving out, and when the liver *qi* is blocked or obstructed then there ceases to be normal circulation, and this can cause irregularity in the period. Either it is too early or too late, or the amount of blood lost is disturbed. If this blockage becomes very serious it can end up creating heat and eventually fire from the internal agitation. The fire exerts a pressure on the blood and its circulation making it irregular and erratic. For example, there can be a lot of very red blood lost in the period.

WOOD AND METAL

Question: We have seen the liver in its relationship to the kidneys and how the liver can go across the *ke* (剋) cycle to affect the stomach and spleen, but we have not talked about how metal affects wood.

Elisabeth Rochat: The first thing to say is that in the emotions which affect the liver we saw that the emotion of grief or oppression, which is the emotion proper to metal and the lungs, was very important. The emotion *you* (憂) has a movement which is the same as that of metal and autumn and the lungs, it collects, gathers together and goes towards concentration. If this movement is too strong it will hinder the opposing movement of the liver. But, on the other hand it will also perfectly balance too great an expansion of outward movement by the liver which could go on expanding indefinitely. In a living person, life is a crossing of these two great movements of springing up and spreading out and gathering in and collecting. In the five movements which create life in the human being and which maintain this life continually, these two great movements which are linked to the liver and to the lungs represent the two great poles of activity. So one can see how they balance each other and how in the case of disturbance there is disharmony and imbalance.

Question: Could you explain more about the physical effect of this control?

Elisabeth Rochat: The physical effect is made through the lungs, because the lungs are the master of *qi*. It is also seen in the relationship between the liver and the breath and its rhythm which are controlled by the lungs. This relationship is an important aspect of the physiology and therefore of the pathology. A weakness in the lung *qi* will have repercussions on the liver *qi* because it will no longer have what is necessary to express itself.

Question: If the metal does not control the wood then the liver fire rises, so is this the reverse *ke* cycle?

Elisabeth Rochat: If there is a weakness in metal there is a weakness in the *qi.* Then there is a lack of efficiency in the springing up of the liver. On the other hand you can have pathological repercussions from the liver onto the lungs. For example, if the liver *qi* is obstructed then this creates fire, and that rises up and seriously injures the lungs. What comes out of this is that the lungs will have lost one of their principal functions which is to clarify and refresh, and to exert a pressure so that things can descend. This is a reverse *ke* cycle, with a pathological effect of the liver affecting the functioning of the lungs with symptoms from the lungs and liver mixed together. For example, you could have coughing, or coughing with blood, pains in the sides and thorax, painful red eyes and a tendency to anger.

THE GALLBLADDER

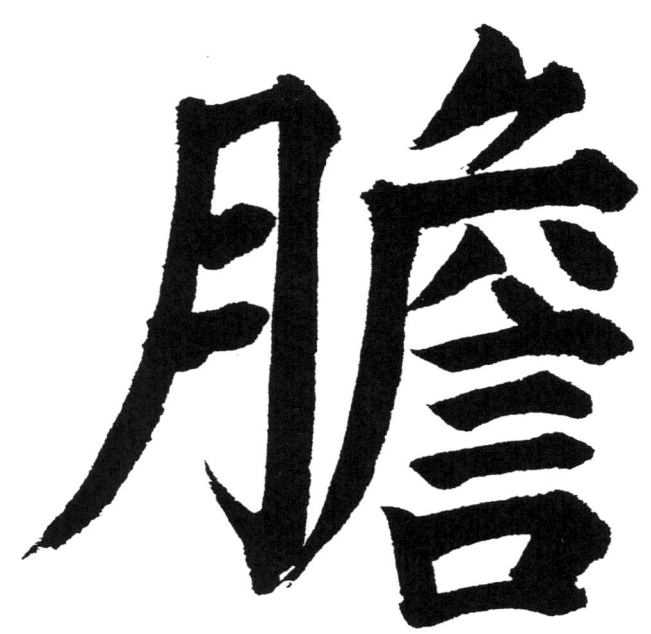

The gallbladder, *dan*

THE GALLBLADDER

Elisabeth Rochat: The charge attributed to the gallbladder in Su wen chapter 8 is to have exactitude, justice and correctness:

> *The gallbladder is responsible for what is just and exact.*
> *Determination and decision stem from it.*

The idea of being just is expressed in the ideogram *zhong* (中) which is also the idea of the centre or median. This character *zhong* often comes up in relationship to the gallbladder, and it is called 'the *fu* (府) of the essences which are in the middle' or 'the *fu* of what is clear and in the middle'. This indicates that the gallbladder is not an ordinary *fu* but an extraordinary *fu*. It is part of the series of the brain, marrow, bones, *mai* (脈), gallbladder and uterus which are referred to as the six extraordinary *fu*. These all have a function of storing essences, or storing the vital code, pattern and basis for all structures of life. In this series only the gallbladder is also one of the six ordinary *fu*, and it therefore has a double role. It is concerned with what is clear and pure, in a manner which is central and which gives exactitude. It works from the interior and, in contrast to the other digestive *fu* it does not have contact with the exterior. Nor is it part of the alimentary canal, so it is not in direct contact with food like the other ordinary *fu*.

Claude Larre: It is like a sort of controller. He is not there on the spot, but he knows everything about the situation. You never see him, but he knows you!

Elisabeth Rochat: It is because of this that the gallbladder has the very elevated, noble position that you see in Su wen chapter 8. It represents the *yang* aspect of the wood, taking decisions and seeing that they are applied without obstacles. The hard strength of the *qi* of *shao yang* (少 陽) makes sure that it can go through any obstruction. The rectitude which exists in the beginning of things ensures that it proceeds in the right way, and that there is no deviation in the way life goes on. It has the idea of something which is very contained, straight and direct. It is for this reason that Su wen chapter 9 says that the eleven *zang* take their decision from the gallbladder.

They need the gallbladder in order to make their decisions, and they consult with it because it has the capacity to give correct judgement. This has an influence on the defence of the whole body and on all the vitality expressed in the *jing shen* (精 神), the vital spirits. The surging up of *qi* could quite easily get out of control, and it needs good direction, like a young child needs a tutor. This is the role of the gallbladder. Therefore it is said that a man who has good gallbladder *qi* is resolute and firmly established, and if his *jing shen* gets over excited or depressed, then the return to normal will be made relatively quickly and easily. Conversely if a man's gallbladder *qi* is feeble and too loose, then he will be constantly subject to illnesses and disturbances. He will never feel well. A symptom of an emptiness of the gallbladder is the tendency to unfounded fears, difficulty in going to sleep calmly and too many dreams. You can also have a bitterness in the mouth, although this can sometimes be a symptom of a fullness of gallbladder *qi*.

As an ordinary *fu* the gallbladder plays a role in facilitating digestion and the absorption of liquids and cereals with the emission of bile, so the loss of this function will have repercussions on the digestion and on the stomach and spleen. You could even have jaundice. Essentially the pathology of the gallbladder as an ordinary *fu* presents with symptoms of heat, for example bitterness in the mouth, dryness in the throat, pains in the thorax and sides, vertigo etc.

Question: I would like to know about the relationship between the gallbladder and the *shen*?

Elisabeth Rochat: The most obvious relationship is that being an extraordinary *fu*, the gallbladder stores essences, and therefore participates in that process which brings the essences to the heart. The essences provide a place for the *shen*, a structure and a means of penetration. The gallbladder also has an intimate relationship with the liver, and is a means of expression for the *hun* and for that which is most *yang* and active. This gives it the ability to make decisions for the eleven other *zang*. It is because of this that it is put in this relationship with the ensemble known as *jing shen*, vital spirits. This is in commentaries later than the Nei jing.

Claude Larre: I am sure that one part of the problem is that in a way the *shen* are more or less under the domination of the *jing*. I mean that if you are able to concentrate enough *jing* you are sending out a call to the *shen*, and they will come in response. While you have to say that the *shen* are free, at the same time you also have to say that they like to come when they are called. We have the same thing in Christianity with the problem of grace. If you do what you are supposed to do then some sort of good or benevolence comes to you. It would come freely, but it is asked for.

There is true friendship between *jing* and *shen*. Not only that, but in the very ordinary texts of Huainan zi it states that the final aim of all human life is to be a companion of the *dao* (道) so if that is the goal the means must follow the same pattern. We have to be friendly with the *shen*, and there has to be a purifying of our essences.

INJURIES TO THE GALLBLADDER

Elisabeth Rochat: When the gallbladder is attacked or injured by outside influences, or by internal attacks coming from the seven emotions, the results can be seen in its dual role as ordinary and extraordinary *fu*. The gallbladder is strong and straight, exact, robust and firm. It knows what is just and correct, and it is determined and resolute. It also has the same quality as the *qi* of *shao yang* which has the strength of beginnings. But it is also the pivot or hinge between different levels in the body. It is said that the *shao yang* is the hinge between the face turned to the exterior and the face turned to the interior, like two sides of a coin, one being a manifestation of the other.

Claude Larre: Exterior and interior are larger concepts than the sides of a coin! That which is inside the human movement of my own personal life may be manifest but not seen. What is not seen is still constructed, and this is called *li* (裡). Although the *li* is not seen it is being built from the time of conception to the time of death. But it does manifest itself and can be seen, and this is the *biao* (表).The *biao* is closer to the exterior, while the structure, *li*, is closer to the interior, so we can refer to them as exterior and interior, but we should really think of them as *biaoli*.

Peter Firebrace: There is a difference between interior and exterior as *nei* (内) and *wai* (外), and as *biao* and *li*. It is quite difficult to find an example of English equivalents. It has been described as the two sides of a coin, and it is definitely not the same as inside and outside.

Elisabeth Rochat: Interior and exterior are rather the definition of two realms, two domains or spheres which can be found at all levels. *Biaoli* is the definition of a passage, something that will turn towards the interior or towards the exterior. *Biao* is made in order to show the effects on the exterior, and *li* is made to reinforce the vitality on the interior. It is exactly the same thing as in paired meridians which show the two sides of an element. It is never said that the two meridians are in the relationship of *neiwai* (内外), interior and exterior, but they are always described as being in the relationship of *biaoli*, showing on the exterior the effects of the element, and then coming back into the interior in order to build the structure of life in the interior.

When the gallbladder is attacked by fire, which is the external attack to which it is most prone and sensitive, then you have symptoms of heat and cold which come and go because of its position as a hinge. The role of the gallbladder as a hinge is because it is both an ordinary and an extraordinary *fu*. It is both that which makes the bile flow and that which stores and treasures the very pure, clear essences. It is a *fu* (府) which has the function of a *zang* (臟).

In the realm of emotions it is above all an emptiness of the gallbladder which is most significant, and which affects its most noble function of storing the pure essences, *jing* (精). This, therefore, influences the vitality which is expressed through the *jing* and *shen*. When the gallbladder is empty there is a kind of fear and apprehension which dominates the person because the movement which should be pushing forward is deficient. There will be accompanying symptoms such as insomnia, madness, blurred vision and bitterness in the mouth. The function of giving a good direction to life is disturbed.

Of course if the liver is dysfunctional it will have an effect on the gallbladder. For example, blockages in the liver *qi* would prevent the transmission of bile, and we would have all the symptoms which are classified under the *yang* of the liver being too strong.

The gallbladder can also be linked in pathology with the stomach and spleen. For example, humidity and heat attacking the spleen can have repercussions on the gallbladder and give rise to certain kinds of jaundice. If there is irregular eating, or eating and drinking too quickly or too much, or if the food is too greasy or there is too much alcohol, all this will give rise to the formation of phlegm and obstruction in the middle heater. These blockages will then have repercussions on the liver and gallbladder and on the circulation of qi and the transmission of bile. All this will give rise to a general congestion which implicates the liver, gallbladder, stomach and spleen. Pains in the ribs can be explained by the pathway of the gallbladder meridian. These pains normally appear when there is blockage in the qi which prevents its spreading out and thus causes pain. The pain can be intermittent, or it can start as not very severe and then become more intense. When the pain is due to stagnation of blood it does not move around and is sharp as a needle. Swellings in the ribs often accompany pains in the ribs, and they can often precede the pain. When this symptom gets worse it can reach the top of the body, the thorax and diaphragm. Below it can affect the whole region of the lower abdomen.

SYNDROMES OF THE LIVER AND GALLBLADDER

LIVER QI OBSTRUCTED AND KNOTTED

gan qi yu jie

肝
氣
郁
結

Elisabeth Rochat: When the liver *qi* is in a state of obstruction or blockage it can form knots *(jie* 結) which means that it cannot spread out correctly. There are five principal categories within this:

1) Blockage of the liver qi within the liver meridian itself

The symptoms here are swelling and pain in the region of the ribs, with pains that can be very deep inside and cannot be located exactly. There is oppression in the region of the thorax, with a tendency to take deep breaths in order to free the sensation of stagnation. For women there can be swollen or painful breasts and irregular periods.

The cause of this could be that the emotions have become imbalanced and no longer enjoy free circulation and harmony. There will be a tendency to anger in this case. There are also repercussions on the pathway of the meridian in the region of the ribs and thorax, and the sensation of oppression. This is particularly present in the thorax because this area is very much involved in the free circulation of the emotions.

When the liver *qi* loses its free circulation then the blood can no longer circulate freely either. It is because of this that you have irregularity in menstruation because of the effect on the functioning of *chong* and *ren mai. Chong* and *ren mai* and the liver are very much involved in the good circulation of blood, particularly in the lower heater.

2) Phlegm and qi cause obstructions and knots

Another aspect of this stagnation of the liver *qi* can be the sensation of having an obstruction in the throat or pharynx, such that you have problems swallowing. It is sometimes called 'globus hystericus'. There is an obstruction at the level of the throat so that the *qi* cannot flow freely through the region of the neck. The blockage of the liver *qi* has repercussions on the functions of the spleen and stomach, and in particular on the spleen's ability to transport and transform, and this leads to the formation of phlegm. If the spleen is not strong enough to transport and transform then there arises a humid, damp stagnation, and added to the obstruction of the liver *qi* already present it creates phlegm.

3) Liver obstructed, qi blocked, blood stagnation

In this case as well as the familiar symptoms of liver *qi* stagnation you will have a darkened complexion, and there can be a tendency to emaciation. In the ribs which are congested and swollen you may also get sharp pains. The liver and spleen will be swollen and the tongue could be dark red or purple, and the sides of the tongue could appear bruised, which is a sign of stagnation. This happens when the blockage of liver *qi* has been present for a long time and there has been such a slowing down in the flow of blood that it has lead to an actual stoppage.

4) Liver qi attacks the stomach

In this case, in addition to all the usual symptoms of liver *qi* stagnation, you have specific pain and swelling in the stomach area. There will also be a tendency to eat less, to have hiccups, eructations or even acid regurgitation because of the weakening of the function of the stomach. The congestion of liver *qi* leads to a blockage in the stomach cavity with pain and swelling there. This is called a transverse countercurrent.

5) Liver qi attacks the spleen

If the blockage in the liver *qi* attacks the spleen then apart from all the expected symptoms you can also get symptoms specifically connected with the spleen such as swelling and pain in the abdomen, gurgling in the intestines and diarrhoea. If you look at the tongue you can often see that it is white and greasy. This is called 'the wood overriding the earth', and it means that the spleen loses its ability to transform and transport. It can no longer conserve and raise the *qi* and that gives rise to the swelling and congestion in the abdomen. The diarrhoea comes from the loss of the function of processing and transforming food correctly, and the inability to control the humidity of the body. In diarrhoea the function of raising things up is completely lost!

When the earth is weak you can also have a deficiency of liver blood because there is an insufficient supply of the materials necessary to renew the essences of the middle heater which go to create blood.

LIVER FIRE BLAZES UPWARDS
gan huo shang yan

肝
火
上
炎

Elisabeth Rochat: This is a fullness of fire in the liver meridian, and in this case you have symptoms such as headaches, blurred vision, vertigo, buzzing in the ears, agitation, tendency to anger, and red face. The pain in the ribs will be burning, and there can be a dryness and bitter taste in the mouth. If these symptoms get worse you can have spitting or vomiting of blood or nosebleed. The urine will be yellow and there can be constipation. There can be quite acute pathology with this situation.

DAMP HEAT IN THE LIVER AND GALLBLADDER
gan dan shi re

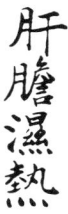

肝
膽
濕
熱

Elisabeth Rochat: This can come from the spleen, so it is a pathology which we often see with the spleen, in particular with the appearance of a certain kind of jaundice. There will be congestion linked with the meridians of the liver and gallbladder, and there may be swelling and pain in the thorax and sides. In the lower *jiao* a man may have swollen, painful testicles and a woman may have a yellow, foul-smelling discharge or pruritus.

COLD BLOCKS THE LIVER NETWORK
han zhi gan mai

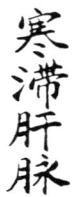

Elisabeth Rochat: The only time cold attacks the liver is by blocking the life-giving network by which the liver can make things circulate. This is especially so in the lower abdomen where the symptoms start off, for example in connection with certain functions of *ren mai*. As you know the liver meridian encircles and goes through the genital region, and is the meridian which is principally concerned with this area. So the lower abdomen will be painful and swollen, the testicles are not held in place properly and tend to be lowered. They will also have a sensation of cold, with a contraction at the level of the scrotum, all of which is caused by cold invading the liver meridian.

LIVER WIND MOVES INSIDE
gan feng nei dong

肝
風
内
動

Elisabeth Rochat: When we speak of wind in the liver we mean internal wind, which is to say the disorder which leads to cramps, muscular contractions, trembling, numbness and paralysis. There are three different causes for this wind:

1) Liver yang transforms into wind

This is when the *yang* of the liver is too strong, often because of a deficiency in the *yin*. With this you get blurred vision, vertigo, dizziness, headache with the feeling of an iron band around the head, numbness and trembling, difficulty speaking and walking. When this is pushed to an extreme you can have apoplexy with a stiff tongue and the mouth and eye deviated. It is also possible to have hemiplegia following this kind of attack by wind. It often comes from the deficiency of *yin* leading to excess fire which disturbs the upper parts of the body. The wind and fire are carried upwards and that is why you get vertigo and headaches, and even difficulties in movement and speech. There is no longer any mastery of movement, and this can be linked to the functioning of the gallbladder which in one part of the Su wen is linked particularly to speech and to that part of the throat.

On the other hand if the movement of the wind cramps the muscles, there is no longer the flexibility that is necessary for the formation of words. If all the strength of the body and the *qi* is carried towards the top because the base and the *yin* is out of balance and is insufficient to pull it downwards, then there will be symptoms of emptiness in the lower part of the body, such as not being able to walk properly.

In addition the fire which is disturbed by the wind will burn up the interstitial fluids, producing phlegm. This will affect the head and orifices of the face, where only the more pure and clear essences should be found.

Following this there can also be a sudden loss of consciousness. If the phlegm flows in the pathways of *qi* this can create terrible disorder, reversing the current's flow and ending in facial distortion and possible hemiplegia with a sudden and violent onset due to the blockage of circulation in one part of the body. In the end there can be cerebral vascular attacks, strokes and so on.

2) *Extreme heat produces wind*

The second possibility for the production of internal wind is by extreme heat, with high fever and great thirst. The person will be disturbed and agitated, with cramps in the limbs and a stiffening of the neck. The muscles of the back and neck will be attacked and arched backwards, the tongue is deviated and agitated by trembling, and there is confusion of consciousness and even delirium. This heat attacks all the systems by which the liver maintains its relations, and of course has a direct effect on the *xin bao luo* (心 包 絡), the network of relationships around the heart which has a special link with the liver. At this point the spirits of the heart can no longer radiate as they should, and the unity and wisdom of the person is damaged creating disturbance. There is a barrier which prevents the *shen* communicating with the interior and which leads to confusion in the mind. It is this which can lead to loss of consciousness.

Heat has a definite effect on all the body fluids which leads to fever and thirst, and as the heat goes deeper and deeper it injures the pathway of the body fluids which should irrigate the muscles leading to the symptoms of cramping and stiffening of the muscles. The muscles and the *jin mai* (筋 脈) lose their nutrition and are subjected to the action of the wind which puts them into spasms and cramps. This can lead to all kinds of different symptoms such as convulsions.

3) Emptiness of blood produces wind

The third manner by which liver wind is produced is from an emptiness of blood. Here again you may have dizziness or vertigo and blurred vision. The complexion will be sallow and withered, and the tongue is often pale with very little coating. The forearms may be numb or you may have sudden and violent cramps, especially in the hands and feet. It is this lack of irrigation which makes the limbs feel impotent, and the absence of liquid support allows the wind to rise up leading to very sudden and violent cramps. The hands and feet are particularly prone because they are at the end of the pathways of irrigation, so it is there that the deficiency is most clearly seen. The cause of this deficiency of the liver blood can be in the kidneys or the spleen, but the blood can no longer nourish the liver, and therefore the liver can no longer nourish what it is responsible for so you have blurred vision and problems in the *jin mai*. There is no great rising up of liver *yang* in this case, rather you have anaemia and chronic illnesses with severe weakening.

EMPTINESS OF LIVER YIN
gan yin xu

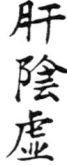

The symptoms of emptiness of liver *yin* can, for greater convenience, be presented in three stages of increasing seriousness:

1) Emptiness of liver blood

The symptoms are dull, lifeless complexion, blurred vision with dizziness; excessive dreaming; buzzing in the ears like cicadas; dry eyes, vision blurred or diminished in the dark; limbs numb or paralysed with spasms in the *jin mai*, the tendinomuscular meridians which run through and stimulate the musculature; flesh quivering with little shivers; nails dull; small quantity of blood in menstruation or amenorrhea. The tongue is pale and the pulse thin, *xi* (細).

The quantity of blood at the body's disposal is small. This situation can arise from a weakness in the production of blood by the spleen and stomach, from a substantial loss of blood or from a long illness. Any of these causes will mean that the quantity of blood stored by the liver is small. The consequences are seen at various levels in the body where the animating power of the liver is important.

In the face, the blood is not abundant enough to give its radiance to the complexion and ensure its rich colouring; nor is it abundant enough to maintain either the irrigation of the eye, which becomes dry, or the clarity and power of vision of the inner system of the eye, so leading to visual disturbances. The nourishment of the brain, which is rich in essence and *yin*, is also diminished, leading to vertigo. The liver meridian makes a direct connection with the inner system of the eye, but through its association with the gallbladder meridian, the *shao yang* of the foot, the ear can also suffer the consequences of the insufficiency of blood. This can lead to noises in the ears, the shrillness indicating the deficiency of blood. One final orifice on the face is affected, the tongue, which is not sufficiently filled with blood to present as a normal red colour and so is pale.

At the extremities of the limbs, the nails, which manifest the muscular force and the inner richness of the liver, are dull since they are poorly nourished. In the layers of the flesh and the pathways which bring them moisture and nutrition, the absence of liver blood gives rise to internal wind. This is responsible for the agitation and quivering of the flesh, muscular spasms and paralysis through blockage due to the erratic movements of the wind.

In women, the liver can no longer provide enough liquid for the periods.

At night, the blood is not sufficient enough to keep the *hun* in their place to control and balance their power of flight and imagination, leading to excessive and doubtless rather agitated dreaming.

The blood which is not available for the liver is also lacking in the whole network of animation, the *mai* (脈). This is shown in the pulse which is thin, *xi* (細).

All treatment will aim to increase and tonify the liver blood.

2) Emptiness of liver yin

In addition to the symptoms given above for emptiness of liver blood, there is an aggravation in the form of internal heat. This internal heat is a result of the empty *yin*. It manifests, most often, as a redness in the cheeks, 'robber sweats' (night time sweating that stops on awakening), insomnia, agitation and malaise in the cardiac region, untimely sweats.

The tongue is red with little coating; the pulse is wiry or bow string (*xian* 弦), thin (*xi* 細), and fast (*shuo* 數).

The agitation of the liver *yang* is created by the lack of blood and the emptiness of *yin;* it affects the fire of the heart, the calm of the spirits, by increasing the heat at the periphery and carrying the circulation away to the exterior, thus causing sweats.

Treatment must increase the *yin* and nourish the liver.

3) Following emptiness of yin the yang is too strong

From a situation of empty liver *yin*, inflammation develops; the rise of internal heat transforms into an internal fire which attacks the kidney *yin* and gives rise to new symptoms. The head and eyes are swollen and painful, vertigo and problems with eyesight intensify and present secondary *yang* characteristics. The noises in the ears are stronger and resemble those which come from an emptiness of kidney *yin*. The limbs are numb and paralysed through absence of blood and the liquids necessary to nourish and move the muscles.

It is a situation called 'extreme emptiness of the trunk and secondary fullness of the branches'. Thus the tongue is red, with a thin yellow coating, indicating internal heat and attack of liquids and *yin*. The pulse is wiry or bowstring (*xian* 弦), and hard (*jian* 堅), indicating the inflammatory attack. The aim of treatment will be to increase the *yin*, balance the liver and reduce the *yang*.

These three levels of illness present a certain number of points in common, but also specific points which make them recognisable and so guide the fundamental principles of treatment. In the first stage, emptiness of liver blood, it is essential to tonify the liver blood. In the second stage, emptiness of liver *yin*, it is important to nourish the liver but also to reinforce the *yin* in a more general way, watching the rise of the heat so as to eventually counter it.

In the third stage, where the *yang* is too strong through emptiness of *yin,* if one wants to try to increase the *yin* and re-establish the balance of the blood and liquids, the first thing to do is to reduce the surging of the liver and weaken the wind. Certain symptoms of the third stage are the same as for the rising of fire in the liver meridian, a direct symptom of perverse fullness. The circumstances of the onset of the illness are generally enough to establish the correct diagnosis.

When the *yang* is too strong due to emptiness of the *yin,* the onset is relatively gradual and there is normally redness of the cheeks and other signs of internal heat. While in the case of fire in the liver meridian the onset is faster and the illness more violent, and there are at the same time signs of full heat, such as the dark colour of the urine.

APPENDIX

THE LIVER AND GALLBLADDER
FROM THE NEIJING JINGYI

THE LIVER

The liver is located under the ribs; its meridian has a connection (*luo* 絡) to the gallbladder; it has the relationship of *biaoli* interior/exterior, with the gallbladder. Among the parts of the body it is linked with the muscles; its orifice opens at the eye.

Its functions are to govern storage and depositing, to regulate the blood of the whole body and to govern the movements of the muscular and bony articulations.

In the regulation of the emotions and the mind, *jing shen qing zhi* (精 神 情 志) the heart plays the role of the central pivot and master, but this regulation is also closely related to the function of the liver.

1)   The liver has the office of general of the armed forces jiang jun (將 軍) *from this comes assessment of circumstances and conception of plans*

The liver, by nature, likes whatever is progressive and lively and dislikes whatever is melancholy and causes obstruction; it corresponds to the *qi* which initiates the upsurging of life, that of spring.

To be in good condition, the liver *qi* must not be either obstructed, withdrawn or full of melancholy, but neither must it be too strong.

If the liver *qi* is excessive, the *yang* rises too strongly and one is agitated and easily angered. If on the other hand, the liver *qi* is insufficient and loses the male force that characterizes its nature, then one is timid and fearful.

In pathology the aspect presented by these illnesses is directly related to the regulatory function of the liver on the emotions and the mind. Agitation, the tendency to anger, fear, timidity - all this follows from loss of the normal functioning of the liver, which gives it the office of the general of the armed forces; this has repercussions on the normal movement of the emotions and the mind and prevents the ability to analyse deeply or to conceive plans with consideration.

2) The liver stores blood
gan cang xue 肝 藏 血

The liver's function of storing (*cang* 藏) the blood is to be differentiated from the heart's function of mastering the life-giving network of the blood (*xue mai* 血 脈). That the liver stores the blood shows the regulation of the quantity of the blood supply. That the heart masters the *xue mai* shows the motive force for the circulation of the blood supply.

The quantity of blood that circulates in the life-giving network (*mai* 脈) is a function of the body's activity, with, in addition, the influences of the *qi* of the four seasons, day and night, *yin* and *yang*; this quantity varies, increasing or decreasing accordingly.

When engaging in activity, the quantity of blood in each part of the body must be increased. But when one is at rest or asleep there is less movement and one then needs less blood; the excess blood then returns to the liver where it is stored.

So, Su wen chapter 10 says:

> *When man is at rest the blood returns to the liver*
> *ren wo xue gui gan* 人 臥 血 歸 肝

If the liver is affected and loses its function of storing the blood, then one can have numerous dreams, be easily frightened and not sleep well. These are symptoms of what is described as the *hun* not being well housed.

3) The liver masters the muscular forces (jin 筋)
it flourishes in the nails

The muscles rely on the bony articulations; contraction and relaxation are the movements of the articulations linked to the bones. When a movement lasts too long or is too violent, then the muscular strength decreases and runs out and one gets tired. If that gets worse, the muscles are injured and can no longer flex or extend.

Su wen chapter 23 says:

> *Walking for a long time injures the muscular forces*
> *jiu xing shang jin* 久 行 傷 筋

Movement is the role of the muscles but the nutrition and maintenance of the muscles originates in the liver. The liver diffuses the essences (*jing* 精) to nourish and maintain the muscles; when the muscles are well maintained, movement can be made with strength.

Su wen chapter 21 says:

> *The vital qi of solid food enters the stomach, there is*
> *diffusion of the essences (jing* 精) *to the liver, there is*
> *impregnation of the qi into the muscles (jin* 筋)

And Su wen chapter 5 says:

The liver masters the muscular forces

But if the liver *qi* is weakened, it cannot supply the muscles with what is necessary for their perfect and full maintenance; then the muscular movements are reduced in strength. For example an old man has slow movements, without skill or flexibility; this is related to the fact that the liver no longer nourishes the muscles.

Su wen chapter 1 says:

In a man of seven times eight years the liver qi declines gan qi shuai 肝 氣 衰

the tendons and muscles are no longer capable of moving jin bu neng dong 筋 不 能 動

The nails are the surplus of the muscles and the muscles are invigorated (*sheng* 生) or produced by the liver. The state of emptiness or fullness of the liver is reflected in the nails.

When the strength of the muscles is robust and vigorous, the nails are very solid. When the muscles are without strength, the nails are very thin and soft. When the liver is ill, the nails are often brittle, dry, dull or change in shape.

Su wen chapter 10 says:

> *The reunion of the liver is in the muscles*
> *gan zhi he jin ye* 肝 之 合 筋 也
> *Its radiance is in the nails*

And again in Su wen chapter 9:

> *The liver is the trunk for extreme cessation (cessation*
> *due to the reaching of an extremity)*
> *gan zhe ba ji zhi ben* 肝 者 罷 極 之 本
>
> *Its flourishing aspect is in the nails*
> *qi hua zai zhao* 其 華 在 爪
>
> *Its full power is in the muscles*
> *qi chong zai jin* 其 充 在 筋
>
> *It is for the production (invigoration) of blood and qi*
> *yi sheng xue qi* 以 生 血 氣

THE GALLBLADDER

The gallbladder is the *fu* (府) of the liver; it stores (*cang* 藏) internally essential juices (*jing zhi* 精 汁). Its meridian has a connection (*luo* 絡) with the liver.

The Nanjing difficulty 49 says:

> *The gallbladder is located between the short leaves of the liver, it is full of essential juices, three hundredths of a bushel.*

Therefore, what are stored in the gallbladder are the essential juices; it is for this reason that Ling shu chapter 2 calls it:

> *the fu of central essences*
> *zhong jing zhi fu* 中 精 之 府

The essences stored in the gallbladder are the clear pure juices (*qing jing* 清 精), quite different from the cloudy (*zhuo* 濁) substances that fill the *fu* and that are for transport and transformation (*chuan hua zhi fu* 傳 化 之 府). These are the *fu* that transport and transform in the digestive tract. This is why the Qiangying yaofang calls it:

> *the fu of central clarity*
> *zhong qing zhi fu* 中 清 之 府

Owing to this characteristic of the gallbladder to store essences (*cang jing* 藏 精) it belongs to the six *fu* (*liu fu* 六 府), but it also belongs to the extraordinary and permanent *fu* (*qi heng zhi fu* 奇 恆 之 府).

The nature of the gallbladder is to be hard and straight. Being hard it is brave and robust, resolute and determined. So the Su wen chapter 8 can say:

> *The gallbladder is responsible for what is just and exact*
> *from it come determination and decision*

The role of the gallbladder is determination and decision. It provides protection against anything that can unduly agitate the *jing shen* (精 神), the essences and spirits, such as great shocks (*da jing* 大 驚) or sudden fears (*cu kong* 卒 恐).

It maintains and controls the normal circulation of *qi* and blood; it keeps the relationship between the different organs harmonious and well-balanced. Its role is therefore very important.

When the *jing shen* (精 神) are agitated, this has repercussions on the normal and healthy functioning of the *zang fu* (藏 府) and can lead to disturbances in the circulation of *qi* and blood.

If the gallbladder *qi* is brave and robust, resolute and firm, then even if the *jing shen* are unduly agitated, causing repercussions and disturbance in the body, these will be of little importance and the return to normal is made relatively quickly.

But if the gallbladder *qi* is weak, there is the opposite condition, which often leads to illness.

INDEX

INDEX